Veterinary Science and Medicine

Veterinary Science and Medicine

Edited by
Kian Churchill

Larsen & Keller
www.larsen-keller.com

Veterinary Science and Medicine
Edited by Kian Churchill
ISBN: 978-1-63549-283-5 (Hardback)

▤ Larsen & Keller

Published by Larsen and Keller Education,
5 Penn Plaza,
19th Floor,
New York, NY 10001, USA

Cataloging-in-Publication Data

Veterinary science and medicine / edited by Kian Churchill.
     p. cm.
Includes bibliographical references and index.
ISBN 978-1-63549-283-5
1. Veterinary medicine. 2. Animals--Diseases. 3. Animal health.
I. Churchill, Kian.
SF745 .V48 2017
636.089--dc23

The publisher's policy is to use permanent paper from mills that operate a sustainable forestry policy. Furthermore, the publisher ensures that the text paper and cover boards used have met acceptable environmental accreditation standards.

Printed and bound in the United States of America.

For more information regarding Larsen and Keller Education and its products, please visit the publisher's website www.larsen-keller.com

Table of Contents

Preface

This book provides comprehensive insights into the field of veterinary science and medicine. It is designed to provide in-depth knowledge about the various concepts and methodologies of this field to the students. Veterinary science refers to that branch of medicinal sciences that is concerned with the diagnosis, prevention and treatment of animals. It deals with the treatment of wild, domestic, and farm animals. The purpose of this text is to provide readers the basic information about this subject. The topics covered in it deal with the fundamental subjects of the area. Some of the themes covered in this book address the varied branches that fall under this category. This textbook is a complete source of knowledge on the present status of this important field.

To facilitate a deeper understanding of the contents of this book a short introduction of every chapter is written below:

Chapter 1- Veterinary medicine is a branch of medicine that helps in the prevention and treatment diseases in animals. It is widely practiced and is also helpful for humans as it monitors and controls zoonotic diseases. The chapter on veterinary medicine offers an insightful focus, keeping in mind the subject matter.

Chapter 2- The various animal vaccines used are anthrax vaccines, DA2PPC vaccines, rabies vaccine, brucellosis vaccine and clostridium vaccines. DA2PP is a vaccine for dogs; it is used to protect them against viruses that are indicated by the alphanumeric characters. The vaccines are given to puppies that are 8 weeks old. The major types of animal vaccines are discussed in this section.

Chapter 3- Equine influenza is the disease that is mainly caused by influenza. A virus that is found in horses. The two main strains of this virus are equine-1 and equine-2. The other types of animal diseases discussed in the chapter are chronic wasting disease, parvovirus, canine transmissible venereal tumor, devil facial tumor disease, skin cancer in horses, panzootic diseases etc. The topics discussed in the chapter are of great importance to broaden the existing knowledge on animal diseases.

Chapter 4- Some of the veterinary drugs mentioned in this section are acepromazine, amitriptyline, boldenone, butorphanol, carprofen, xylazine and neoplasene. Acepromazine is an antipsychotic drug that is used in humans and animals both. This drug is used on animals that are hyperactive or are fractious. The topics discussed in the section are of great importance to broaden the existing knowledge on veterinary drugs.

Chapter 5- Animal euthanasia is the act of putting an animal to death. The usual reasons for euthanasia are incurable diseases or unfortunately the lack of resources. Alternatively, the other veterinary procedures mentioned are dysthanasia, organ replacement in animals, tibial tuberosity advancement and an overview of discretionary invasive procedures on animals. This chapter will provide an integrated understanding of veterinary procedures.

Chapter 6- Onychectomy is the process of surgically declawing any animal. The claw bone is amputated because it develops germinal tissue. This act is practiced in some countries whereas in some countries it is considered to be an act of animal cruelty. The other cosmetic procedures that are performed on animals are docking, cropping and devocalization. The major categories of cosmetic procedures are dealt with great details in the chapter.

Chapter 7- An Elizabethan collar is a medical device that is worn by animals; it is shaped like a cone and its main purpose is to prevent the animal from biting its own body. This is done so that the wound that the animal has is properly healed. Dog crate, nose ring, livestock crush, screw picket, muzzle and elastration are some of the tools and equipments used in veterinary medicine. The aspects elucidated in this chapter are of vital importance, and provide a better understanding of veterinary medicine.

Chapter 8- Veterinary physicians are doctors who practice veterinary medicine by treating animals for their injury or disorders. They usually practice in clinics as well as in outdoors. Some of the other various veterinary professions are paraveterinary workers, equine dentists and animal nutritionists. The chapter explains to the readers the importance of the various veterinary professions.

Chapter 9- Hippiatrica is a collection of the ancient Greek texts that focus on the concern and care shown towards animals, horses in particular. Epizootic and mulomedicina chironis are the alternative topics explained in the chapter. The topics discussed in the section are of great importance to broaden the existing knowledge on the evolution of veterinary science.

I would like to share the credit of this book with my editorial team who worked tirelessly on this book. I owe the completion of this book to the never-ending support of my family, who supported me throughout the project.

Editor

Introduction to Veterinary Medicine

Veterinary medicine is a branch of medicine that helps in the prevention and treatment diseases in animals. It is widely practiced and is also helpful for humans as it monitors and controls zoonotic diseases. The chapter on veterinary medicine offers an insightful focus, keeping in mind the subject matter.

Veterinary medicine is the branch of medicine that deals with the prevention, diagnosis and treatment of disease, disorder and injury in non-human animals. The scope of veterinary medicine is wide, covering all animal species, both domesticated and wild, with a wide range of conditions which can affect different species.

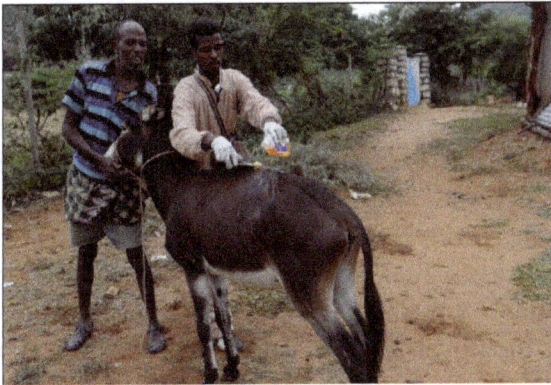

A veterinary technician in Ethiopia shows the owner of an ailing donkey how to sanitize the site of infection.

Veterinary medicine is widely practiced, both with and without professional supervision. Professional care is most often led by a veterinary physician (also known as a vet, veterinary surgeon or veterinarian), but also by paraveterinary workers such as veterinary nurses or technicians. This can be augmented by other paraprofessionals with specific specialisms such as animal physiotherapy or dentistry, and species relevant roles such as farriers.

Veterinary science helps human health through the monitoring and control of zoonotic disease (infectious disease transmitted from non-human animals to humans), food safety, and indirectly through human applications from basic medical research. They also help to maintain food supply through livestock health monitoring and treatment, and mental health by keeping pets healthy and long living. Veterinary scientists often collaborate with epidemiologists, and other health or natural scientists depending on type of work. Ethically, veterinarians are usually obliged to look after animal welfare.

History

Premodern Era

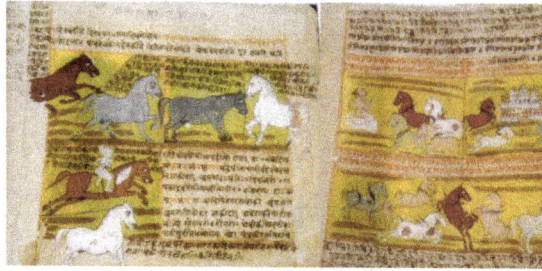

"Shalihotra" manuscript pages

The Egyptian *Papyrus of Kahun* (1900 BCE) and Vedic literature in ancient India offer one of the first written records of veterinary medicine. (Buddhism) First Buddhist Emperor of India edicts of Asoka reads: "Everywhere King Piyadasi (Asoka) made two kinds of medicine medicine for people and medicine for animals. Where there were no healing herbs for people and animals, he ordered that they be bought and planted."

The first attempts to organize and regulate the practice of treating animals tended to focus on horses because of their economic significance. In the Middle Ages from around 475 CE, farriers combined their work in horseshoeing with the more general task of "horse doctoring". In 1356, the Lord Mayor of London, concerned at the poor standard of care given to horses in the city, requested that all farriers operating within a seven-mile radius of the City of London form a "fellowship" to regulate and improve their practices. This ultimately led to the establishment of the Worshipful Company of Farriers in 1674.

Meanwhile, Carlo Ruini's book *Anatomia del Cavallo,* (*Anatomy of the Horse*) was published in 1598. It was the first comprehensive treatise on the anatomy of a non-human species.

Establishment of Profession

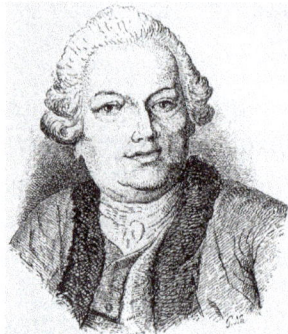

Claude Bourgelat established the earliest veterinary college in Lyon in 1762.

The first veterinary college was founded in Lyon, France in 1762 by Claude Bourgelat. According to Lupton, after observing the devastation being caused by cattle plague to the French herds, Bourgelat devoted his time to seeking out a remedy. This resulted in his founding a veterinary college in Lyon in 1761, from which establishment he dispatched students to combat the disease; in a short time, the plague was stayed and the health of stock restored, through the assistance rendered to agriculture by veterinary science and art."

The Odiham Agricultural Society was founded in 1783 in England to promote agriculture and industry, and played an important role in the foundation of the veterinary profession in Britain. A founding member, Thomas Burgess, began to take up the cause of animal welfare and campaign for the more humane treatment of sick animals. A 1785 Society meeting resolved to "promote the study of Farriery upon rational scientific principles."

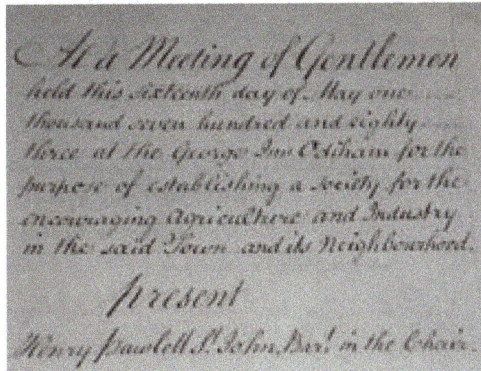

Minutes taken at the establishment of the Odiham Agricultural Society, which went on to play a pivotal role in the establishment of the veterinary profession in England.

The physician James Clark wrote a treatise entitled *Prevention of Disease* in which he argued for the professionalization of the veterinary trade, and the establishment of veterinary colleges. This was finally achieved in 1790, through the campaigning of Granville Penn, who persuaded the Frenchman, Benoit Vial de St. Bel to accept the professorship of the newly established Veterinary College in London. The Royal College of Veterinary Surgeons was established by royal charter in 1844. Veterinary science came of age in the late 19th century, with notable contributions from Sir John McFadyean, credited by many as having been the founder of modern Veterinary research.

In the United States, the first schools were established in the early 19th century in Boston, New York and Philadelphia. In 1879, Iowa Agricultural College became the first land grant college to establish a school of veterinary medicine. Suzanne Saueressig became the first accredited female veterinarian in Missouri in 1955.

Veterinary Physicians

Veterinary care and management is usually led by a veterinary physician (usually called a vet, veterinary surgeon or veterinarian). This role is the equivalent of a doctor in human medicine, and usually involves post-graduate study and qualification.

In many countries, the local nomenclature for a vet is a protected term, meaning that people without the prerequisite qualifications and/or registration are not able to use the title, and in many cases, the activities that may be undertaken by a vet (such as animal treatment or surgery) are restricted only to those people who are registered as vet. For instance, in the United Kingdom, as in other jurisdictions, animal treatment may only be performed by registered vets (with a few designated exceptions, such as paraveterinary workers), and it is illegal for any person who is not registered to call themselves a vet or perform any treatment.

Most vets work in clinical settings, treating animals directly. These vets may be involved in a general practice, treating animals of all types; may be specialized in a specific group of animals such as companion animals, livestock, laboratory animals, zoo animals or horses; or may specialize in a narrow medical discipline such as surgery, dermatology, laboratory animal medicine, or internal medicine.

As with healthcare professionals, vets face ethical decisions about the care of their patients. Current debates within the profession include the ethics of purely cosmetic procedures on animals, such as declawing of cats, docking of tails, cropping of ears and debarking on dogs.

Paraveterinary Workers

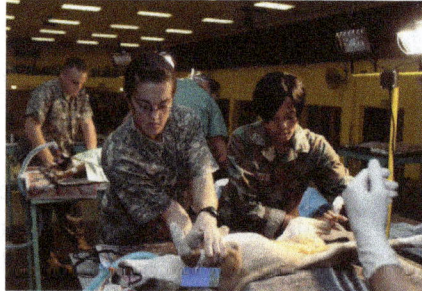

US and South African army veterinary technicians prepare a dog for spaying.

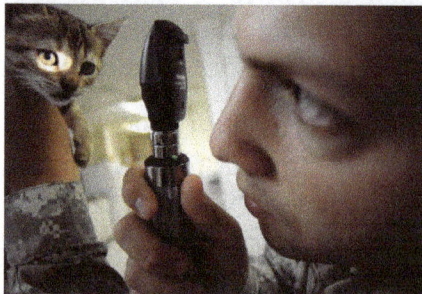

An eye exam of a kitten under way prior to the kitten's adoption.

Paraveterinary workers, including veterinary nurses, technicians and assistants, either assist vets in their work, or may work within their own scope of practice, depending on skills and qualifications, including in some cases, performing minor surgery.

The role of paraveterinary workers is less homogeneous globally than that of a vet, and qualification levels, and the associated skill mix, vary widely.

Allied Professions

A number of professions exist within the scope of veterinary medicine, but which may not necessarily be performed by vets or veterinary nurses. This includes those performing roles which are also found in human medicine, such as practitioners dealing with musculoskeletal disorders, including osteopaths, chiropractors and physiotherapists.

There are also roles which are specific to animals, but which have parallels in human society, such as animal grooming and animal massage.

Some roles are specific to a species or group of animals, such as farriers, who are involved in the shoeing of horses, and in many cases have a major role to play in ensuring the medical fitness of the horse.

Veterinary Research

Veterinary research includes research on prevention, control, diagnosis, and treatment of diseases of animals and on the basic biology, welfare, and care of animals. Veterinary research transcends species boundaries and includes the study of spontaneously occurring and experimentally induced models of both human and animal disease and research at human-animal interfaces, such as food safety, wildlife and ecosystem health, zoonotic diseases, and public policy.

Clinical Veterinary Research

As in medicine, randomized controlled trials are fundamental also in veterinary medicine to establish the effectiveness of a treatment. However, clinical veterinary research is far behind human medical research, with fewer randomized controlled trials, that have a lower quality and that are mostly focused on research animals. Possible improvement consists in creation of network for inclusion of private veterinary practices in randomized controlled trials.

References

- Di Girolamo, N (2016). "Deficiencies of effectiveness of intervention studies in veterinary medicine: a cross-sectional survey of ten leading veterinary and medical journals". PeerJ. 4: e1649. doi:10.7717/peerj.1649.

- Sargeant, JM (2010). "Quality of reporting of clinical trials of dogs and cats and associations with treatment effects.". Journal of veterinary internal medicine. 24 (1): 44–50. doi:10.1111/j.1939-1676.2009.0386.x.

Various Animal Vaccines

The various animal vaccines used are anthrax vaccines, DA2PPC vaccines, rabies vaccine, brucellosis vaccine and clostridium vaccines. DA2PP is a vaccine for dogs; it is used to protect them against viruses that are indicated by the alphanumeric characters. The vaccines are given to puppies that are 8 weeks old. The major types of animal vaccines are discussed in this section.

Anthrax Vaccines

Vaccines against the livestock and human disease anthrax—caused by the bacterium *Bacillus anthracis*—have had a prominent place in the history of medicine, from Pasteur's pioneering 19th-century work with cattle (the first effective bacterial vaccine and the second effective vaccine ever) to the controversial late 20th century use of a modern product to protect American troops against the use of anthrax in biological warfare. Human anthrax vaccines were developed by the Soviet Union in the late 1930s and in the US and UK in the 1950s. The current vaccine approved by the U.S. Food and Drug Administration (FDA) was formulated in the 1960s.

Currently administered human anthrax vaccines include acellular (USA, UK) and live spore (Russia) varieties. All currently used anthrax vaccines show considerable local and general reactogenicity (erythema, induration, soreness, fever) and serious adverse reactions occur in about 1% of recipients. New third-generation vaccines being researched include recombinant live vaccines and recombinant sub-unit vaccines.

Pasteur's Vaccine

In the 1870s, the French chemist Louis Pasteur (1822–1895) applied his previous method of immunizing chickens against chicken cholera to anthrax, which affected cattle, and thereby aroused widespread interest in combating other diseases with the same approach. In May 1881, Pasteur performed a famous public experiment at Pouilly-le-Fort to demonstrate his concept of vaccination. He prepared two groups of 25 sheep, one goat and several cows. The animals of one group were twice injected, with an interval of 15 days, with an anthrax vaccine prepared by Pasteur; a control group was left unvaccinated. Thirty days after the first injection, both groups were injected with a culture of live anthrax bacteria. All the animals in the non-vaccinated group died, while all of the animals in the vaccinated group survived. The public reception was sensational.

Pasteur publicly claimed he had made the anthrax vaccine by exposing the bacilli to oxygen. His laboratory notebooks, now in the Bibliothèque Nationale in Paris, in fact show Pasteur used the method of rival Jean-Joseph-Henri Toussaint (1847–1890), a Toulouse veterinary surgeon, to create the anthrax vaccine. This method used the oxidizing agent potassium dichromate. Pasteur's oxygen method did eventually produce a vaccine but only after he had been awarded a patent on the production of an anthrax vaccine.

The notion of a weak form of a disease causing immunity to the virulent version was not new; this had been known for a long time for smallpox. Inoculation with smallpox (variolation) was known to result in far less scarring, and greatly reduced mortality, in comparison with the naturally acquired disease. The English physician Edward Jenner (1749–1823) had also discovered (1796) the process of vaccination by using cowpox to give cross-immunity to smallpox and by Pasteur's time this had generally replaced the use of actual smallpox material in inoculation. The difference between smallpox vaccination and anthrax or chicken cholera vaccination was that the weakened form of the latter two disease organisms had been "generated artificially", so a naturally weak form of the disease organism did not need to be found. This discovery revolutionized work in infectious diseases and Pasteur gave these artificially weakened diseases the generic name "vaccines", in honor of Jenner's groundbreaking discovery. In 1885, Pasteur produced his celebrated first vaccine for rabies by growing the virus in rabbits and then weakening it by drying the affected nerve tissue.

In 1995, the centennial of Pasteur's death, the *New York Times* ran an article titled "Pasteur's Deception". After having thoroughly read Pasteur's lab notes, the science historian Gerald L. Geison declared Pasteur had given a misleading account of the preparation of the anthrax vaccine used in the experiment at Pouilly-le-Fort. The same year, Max Perutz published a vigorous defense of Pasteur in the *New York Review of Books*.

Sterne's Vaccine

The Austrian-South African immunologist Max Sterne (1905–1997) developed an attenuated live animal vaccine in 1935 that is still employed and derivatives of his strain account for almost all veterinary anthrax vaccines used in the world today. Beginning in 1934 at the Onderstepoort Veterinary Research Institute, north of Pretoria, he prepared an attenuated anthrax vaccine, using the method developed by Pasteur. A persistent problem with Pasteur's vaccine was achieving the correct balance between virulence and immunogenicity during preparation. This notoriously difficult procedure regularly produced casualties among vaccinated animals. With little help from colleagues, Sterne performed small-scale experiments which isolated the "Sterne strain" (34F2) of anthrax which became, and remains today, the basis of most of the improved livestock anthrax vaccines throughout the world.

Russian Anthrax Vaccines

Anthrax vaccines were developed in the Soviet Union in the 1930s and available for use in humans by 1940. A live attenuated, unencapsulated spore vaccine became widely used for humans. It was given either by scarification or subcutaneously and its developers claimed that it was reasonably well tolerated and showed some degree of protective efficacy against cutaneous anthrax in clinical field trials. The efficacy of the live Russian vaccine was reported to have been greater than that of either of the killed British or US anthrax vaccines (AVP and AVA, respectively) during the 1970s and '80s. Today both Russia and China use live attenuated strains for their human vaccines. These vaccines may be given by aerosol, scarification, or subcutaneous injection. A Georgian/Russian live anthrax spore vaccine (called STI) was based on spores from the Sterne strain of *B. anthracis*. It was given in a two-dose schedule, but serious side-effects restricted its use to healthy adults. It was reportedly manufactured at the George Eliava Institute of Bacteriophage, Microbiology and Virology in Tbilisi, Georgia, until 1991.

British Anthrax Vaccines

British biochemist Harry Smith (1921–2011), working for the UK bio-weapons program at Porton Down, discovered the three anthrax toxins in 1948. This discovery was the basis of the next generation of antigenic anthrax vaccines and for modern antitoxins to anthrax. The widely used British anthrax vaccine—sometimes called Anthrax Vaccine Precipitated (AVP) to distinguish it from the similar AVA—became available for human use in 1954. This was a cell-free vaccine in distinction to the live-cell Pasteur-style vaccine previously used for veterinary purposes. It is now manufactured by Porton Biopharma Ltd, a Company owned by the UK Department of Health.

AVP is administered at primovaccination in three doses with a booster dose after six months. The active ingredient is a sterile filtrate of an alum-precipitated anthrax antigen from the Sterne strain in a solution for injection. The other ingredients are aluminium potassium sulphate, sodium chloride and purified water. The preservative is thiomersal (0.005%). The vaccine is given by intramuscular injection and the primary course of four single injections (3 injections 3 weeks apart, followed by a 6-month dose) is followed by a single booster dose given once a year. During the Gulf War (1990–1991), UK military personnel were given AVP concomitantly with the pertussis vaccine as an adjuvant to improve overall immune response and efficacy.

American Anthrax Vaccines

The United States undertook basic research directed at producing a new anthrax vaccine during the 1950s and '60s. The product known as Anthrax Vaccine Adsorbed (AVA)—trade name *BioThrax*—was licensed in 1970 by the U.S. National Institutes of Health (NIH) and in 1972 the Food and Drug Administration (FDA) took over responsibility for vaccine licensure and oversight. AVA is produced from culture filtrates of an avirulent, nonencapsulated mutant of the *B. anthracis* Vollum strain known as V770-NP1-R. No living organisms are present in the vaccine which results in protective immunity after 3 to 6 doses. AVA remains the only FDA-licensed human anthrax vaccine in the United States and is produced by Emergent BioSolutions, formerly known as BioPort Corporation in Lansing, Michigan. The principal purchasers of the vaccine in the United States are the Department of Defense and Department of Health and Human Services. Ten million doses of AVA have been purchased for the U.S. Strategic National Stockpile for use in the event of a mass bioterrorist anthrax attack.

In 1997, the Clinton administration initiated the Anthrax Vaccine Immunization Program (AVIP), under which active U.S. service personnel were to be immunized with the vaccine. Controversy ensued since vaccination was mandatory and a perception developed that AVA was unsafe, causing sometimes serious side effects. Mandatory vaccinations were halted in 2004 by a formal legal injunction which made numerous substantive challenges regarding the vaccine and its safety. After reviewing extensive scientific evidence, the FDA again determined in 2005 that AVA is safe and effective as licensed for the prevention of anthrax, regardless of the route of exposure. In 2006, the Defense Department announced the reinstatement of mandatory anthrax vaccinations for more than 200,000 troops and defense contractors. Despite another lawsuit filed by the same attorneys, the vaccinations are required for most U.S. military units and civilian contractors assigned to homeland bioterrorism defense or deployed in Iraq, Afghanistan or South Korea.

Investigational Anthrax Vaccines

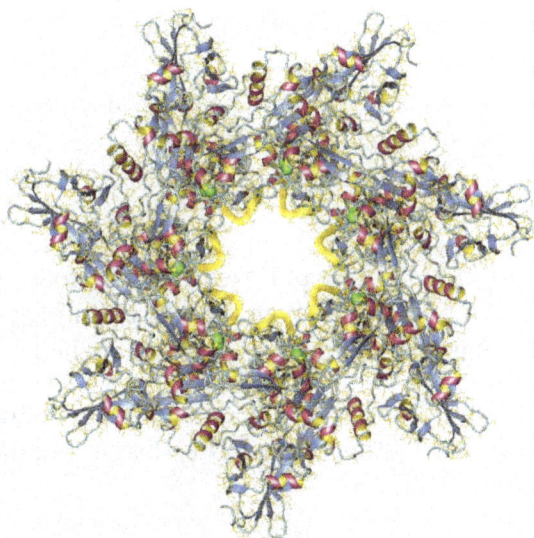

Anthrax toxin protective antigen (fragment) heptamer, *Bacillus anthracis*.

A number of experimental anthrax vaccines are undergoing pre-clinical testing, notably the *Bacillus anthracis* protective antigen—known as PA

- Omer-2 trial: Beginning in 1998 and running for eight years, a secret Israeli project known as *Omer-2* tested an Israeli investigational anthrax vaccine on 716 volunteers of the Israel Defense Forces. The vaccine—given under a seven-dose schedule—was developed by the Nes Tziona Biological Institute. A group of study volunteers complained of multi-symptom illnesses allegedly associated with the vaccine and petitioned for disability benefits to the Defense Ministry, but were denied. In February 2009, a petition from the volunteers to disclose a report about *Omer-2* was filed with the Israel's High Court against the Defense Ministry, the Israel Institute for Biological Research at Nes Tziona, the director, Avigdor Shafferman, and the IDF Medical Corps. Release of the information was requested to support further action to provide disability compensation for the volunteers. In 2014 it was announced that the Israeli government would pay $6 million compensation to the 716 soldiers who participated in the Omer-2 trial.

- In 2012, *B. anthracis* isolate H9401 was obtained from a Korean patient suffering from gastrointestinal anthrax. The goal of the Republic of Korea is to use this strain as a challenge strain to develop a recombinant vaccine against anthrax.

DA2PPC Vaccine

DA2PP, is a multivalent vaccine for dogs that protects against the viruses indicated by the alphanumeric characters forming the acronym: D for canine distemper, A2 for canine adenovirus type 2, which offers cross-protection to canine adenovirus type 1 (the more pathogenic of the two strains), the first P for canine parvovirus, and the second P for parainfluenza. Because infectious canine hepatitis is another name for canine adenovirus type 1, an H is sometimes used instead of A. In DA2PPC, the C indicates canine coronavirus.

This vaccine is usually given to puppies at 8 weeks of age, followed by 12 weeks of age, and then 16 weeks of age. This vaccine is given again at 1 year of age and then annually, or every 3 years. Some veterinarians' recommended vaccine schedules may differ from this.

DA2PPC does not include Bordetella. But the combination of Bordetella with DA2PPC prevents kennel cough, by preventing adenovirus, distemper, parainfluenza, and Bordetella.

For Distemper

While the DA2PPC vaccine also protects against parainfluenza, parvovirus, adenovirus, and canine coronavirus, it most importantly protects against the debilitating and deadly disease canine distemper, an often fatal viral illness that causes neurologic dysfunction, pneumonia, nonspecific systemic symptoms such as fever and fatigue, and weight loss, as well as upper respiratory symptoms and diarrhea, poor appetite, and vomiting. There is no antiviral drug effective against the canine distemper virus. Treatment is supportive and consists of antibiotics to prevent secondary infections, anticonvulsants for seizures, and intravenus fluids to prevent dehydration. Given the lethality of distemper and the relative rarity of side effects from the vaccine, all reputable veterinarians recommend the DA2PPC vaccine. Also, even if the dog owner is not concerned about adenovirus, coronavirus, parvovirus, or parainfluenza, they should vaccinate their dogs to protect them against distemper.

DHPP, DAPP, DA2PP, and DAPPC are not the same. The names are often used interchangeably but they are different. Distemper, adenovirus type 1 (thus hepatitis), parainfluenza, and parvovirus are covered by all 4. DHPP covers adenovirus type 1 and may or may not cover adenovirus type 2. And only DAPPC covers coronavirus.

DAPP or DA2PP are the most commonly used. Coronavirus has not been proven to cause any significant disease in dogs so it is a useless vaccine.

Rabies Vaccine

Rabies vaccine is a vaccine used to prevent rabies. There are a number of vaccines available that are both safe and effective. They can be used to prevent rabies before and for a period of time after exposure to the virus such as by a dog or bat bite. The immunity that develops is long lasting after three doses. Doses are usually given by injection into the skin or muscle. After exposure vaccination is typically used along with rabies immunoglobulin. It is recommended that those who are at high risk of exposure be vaccinated before potential exposure. Vaccines are effective in humans and other animals. Vaccinating dogs is very effective in preventing the spread of rabies to humans.

Rabies vaccines may be safely used in all age groups. About 35 to 45 percent of people develop a brief period of redness and pain at the injection site. About 5 to 15 percent of people may have fever, headaches, or nausea. After exposure to rabies there is no contraindication to its use. Most vaccines do not contain thimerosal. Vaccines made from nerve tissue are used in a few countries, mainly in Asia and Latin America, but are less effective and have greater side effects. Their use is thus not recommended by the World Health Organization.

The first rabies vaccine was introduced in 1885, which was followed by an improved version in 1908. Millions of people globally have been vaccinated and it is estimated that this saves more than 250,000 people a year. It is on the World Health Organization's List of Essential Medicines, the most important medication recommended for a basic health system. The wholesale cost in the developing world is between 44 and 78 USD for a course of treatment as of 2014. In the United States a course of rabies vaccine is more than 750 USD.

Medical Uses

The World Health Organization recommends vaccinating in those who are at high risk of the disease including children who live in areas where it is common. Four doses are given over a one-month period.

Additional Doses

Immunity following a course of doses is typically long lasting. Additional doses are not typically needed except in those at very high risk. Following administration of a booster dose, one study found 97% of immuno-competent individuals demonstrate protective levels of neutralizing antibodies at 10 years.

Types

The human diploid cell rabies vaccine (H.D.C.V.) was started in 1967. Human diploid cell rabies vaccines are inactivated vaccines made using the attenuated Pitman-Moore L503 strain of the virus. Human diploid cell rabies vaccines have been given to more than 1.5 million people as of 2006.

In addition to these developments, newer and less expensive purified chicken embryo cell vaccine, and purified Vero cell rabies vaccine are now available. The purified Vero cell rabies vaccine uses the attenuated Wistar strain of the rabies virus, and uses the Vero cell line as its host.

History

Virtually every infection with rabies resulted in death until two French scientists, Louis Pasteur and Émile Roux, developed the first rabies vaccination in 1885. This vaccine was first used on a human on July 6, 1885, on nine-year-old Joseph Meister (1876–1940), who had been mauled by a rabid dog.

Their vaccine consisted of a sample of the virus harvested from infected (and necessarily dead) rabbits, which was weakened by allowing it to dry for 5 to 10 days. Similar nerve tissue-derived vaccines are still used now in some countries, and while they are much cheaper than modern cell culture vaccines, they are not as effective. Neural tissue vaccines also carry a certain risk of neurological complications.

Other Animals

Aside from vaccinating humans, another approach was also developed by vaccinating dogs to prevent the spread of the virus. In 1979 the Van Houweling Research Laboratory of the Silliman University Medical Center in Dumaguete in the Philippines, then headed by Dr. George Beran, developed and produced a dog vaccine that gave a three-year immunity from rabies. The development of the vaccine resulted in the elimination of rabies in many parts of the Visayas and Mindanao Islands. The successful program in the Philippines was later used as a model by other countries, such as Ecuador and the Yucatan State of Mexico, in their fight against rabies conducted in collaboration with the World Health Organization.

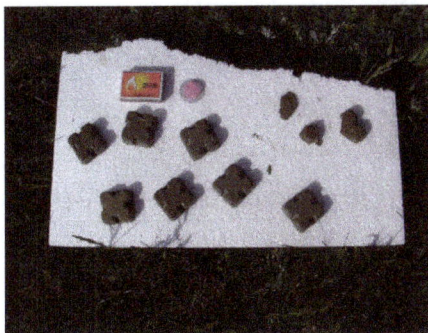

Baits with vaccine for oral vaccination

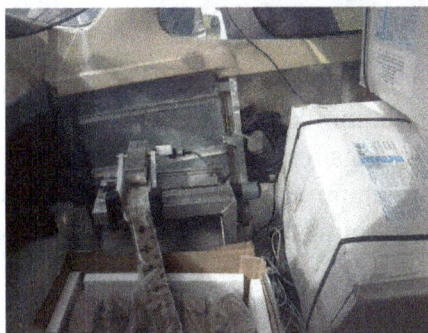

Machine for distribution of baits from airplane

In Tunisia a rabies control program was initiated to give dog owners free vaccination to promote mass vaccination which was sponsored by their government. The vaccine is known as Rabisin (Mérial), which is a cell based rabies vaccine only used countrywide. Vaccinations are often administered when owners take in their dogs for check-ups and visits at the vet.

Pre-exposure immunization has been used on domesticated and wild populations. In many jurisdictions, domestic dogs, cats, ferrets, and rabbits are required to be vaccinated.

There is also vaccination in pellet form which can be left out for wild animals to produce a herd immunity effect. Oral vaccination against rabies is a preventive measure to eradicate rabies in wild animals, vectors of disease, mainly foxes, raccoons, raccoon dogs, coyotes and jackals, but also can be used for dogs in developing countries. Baits are distributed by airplanes in rural areas and by hand in urban and suburban areas.

The idea of wildlife vaccination was conceived during the 1960s, and modified-live rabies viruses were used for the experimental oral vaccination of carnivores by the 1970s. The development of safe and effective rabies virus vaccines applied in attractive baits resulted in the first field trials in Switzerland in 1978.

Imrab is an example of a veterinary rabies vaccine containing the Pasteur strain of killed rabies virus. Several different types of Imrab exist, including Imrab, Imrab 3, and Imrab Large Animal. Imrab 3 has been approved for ferrets and, in some areas, pet skunks.

Brucellosis Vaccine

Brucellosis vaccine is a vaccine for cattle, sheep and goats used against brucellosis.

Currently, there is no vaccine available for humans.

Clostridium Vaccine

Hectivac-Pis a vaccine for sheep in the United Kingdom that protects sheep against 7 clostridial diseases and pneumonia. It should be administered subcutaneously at least 4 weeks before lambing. This results in the specific antibodies being produced by B-cells and secreted into the mammary glands. These antibodies in the colostrum of the vaccinated sheep provide immunity to her lambs. Booster injections are required to sustain immunity.

References

- Decker, Janet (2003). Deadly Diseases and Epidemics, Anthrax. Chelesa House Publishers. pp. 27–28. ISBN 0-7910-7302-5.

- See Gerald Geison, The Private Science of Louis Pasteur, Princeton University Press, 1995. ISBN 0-691-01552-X. May 1995 NY Times

- Guillemin, Jeanne (1999). ANTHRAX, the investigation of a Deadly Outbreak. University of California Press. p. 34. ISBN 0-520-22917-7.

- Nunnally, Brian (2014). Vaccine Analysis: Strategies, Principles, and Control. Springer. p. 63. ISBN 9783662450246.

- Shlim, David (June 30, 2015). «Perspectives: Intradermal Rabies Preexposure Immunization». Retrieved 6 December 2015.

- WHO Model List of EssentialMedicines» (PDF). World Health Organization. October 2013. Retrieved 22 April 2014.

- Dr. George W. Beran›s Biography» Archived April 15, 2010, at the Wayback Machine.. World Rabies Day. Retrieved 2010-04-23.

Animal Diseases and its Types

Equine influenza is the disease that is mainly caused by influenza. A virus that is found in horses. The two main strains of this virus are equine-1 and equine-2. The other types of animal diseases discussed in the chapter are chronic wasting disease, parvovirus, canine transmissible venereal tumor, devil facial tumor disease, skin cancer in horses, panzootic diseases etc. The topics discussed in the chapter are of great importance to broaden the existing knowledge on animal diseases.

Equine Influenza

Equine influenza (horse flu) is the disease caused by strains of influenza A that are enzootiin horse species. Equine influenza occurs globally, previously caused by two main strains of virus: equine-1 (H7N7) and equine-2 (H3N8). The OIE now considers H7N7 strains likely to be extinct since these stains have not been isolated for over 20 years. Predominant international circulating H3N8 strains are Florida sublineage of the American lineage; clade 1 predominates in the Americas and clade 2 in Europe. (Elton and Cullinane, 2013; Paillot, 2014; Slater et al., 2013).The disease has a nearly 100% infection rate in an unvaccinated horse population with no prior exposure to the virus.

While equine influenza is historically not known to affect humans, impacts of past outbreaks have been devastating due to the economireliance on horses for communication (postal service), military (cavalry), and general transportation. In modern times, though, the ramifications of equine influenza are most clear in the horse-racing industry.

Characteristics

Equine influenza is characterized by a very high rate of transmission among horses, and has a relatively short incubation time of one to five days. Horses with horse flu can run a fever, have a dry, hacking cough, have a runny nose, and become depressed and reluctant to eat or drink for several days, but they usually recover in two to three weeks.

An 1872 report on equine influenza describes the disease as:

"An epizootispecififever of a very debilitating type, with inflammation of the respiratory mucous membrane, and less frequently of other organs, having an average duration of ten to fifteen days, and not conferring immunity from a second attack in subsequent epizootics."

— James Law, Report of the Commissioner of Agriculture for the year 1872

Causes

Equine influenza is caused by several strains of the influenza A virus endemito horses. Viruses that cause equine influenza were first isolated in 1956. They can cross the species barrier to cause an epizootidisease in humans, and recently, in dogs.

The equine-1 virus affects heart muscle, while the equine-2 virus is much more severe and systemic. The disease is primarily spread between infected horses. Exposure to infected waste materials (urine and manure) in stables leads to rapid spread of the disease.

History

A comprehensive report describing the disease - compiled in response to the 1872 outbreak of the disease in North America - provided a thorough examination of the history of the disease.

Early Records

The report notes putative cases dating as far back as Hippocrates and Livius. Absyrtus, a Greek veterinarian from 330 CE, described a disease in the horse population having the general characters of influenza, which the report mentions as the earliest clear record of equine influenza in the lower animals.

The report notes the next recorded equine influenza case in 1299, the same year that a catarrhal epidemiaffected Europe. Spanish records noted cases in which "The horse carried his head drooping, would eat nothing, ran from the eyes, and there was hurried beating of the flanks. The malady was epidemic, and in that year one thousand horses died."

Prevalence of influenza is found in historirecords in the centuries of the Middle Ages, but direct implication of horses is not always clear. Neither are recorded instances of record deaths among horses and other animals clear on the exact cause of death.

1872 North American Outbreak

An epizootioutbreak of equine influenza during 1872 in North America became known as "The Great Epizootiof 1872". The outbreak is known as the "most destructive recorded episode of equine influenza in history". In 1870, three-fourths of Americans lived in rural areas (towns under 2500 population, and farms). Horse and mule power was used for moving wagons and carriages, and pulling plows and farm equipment. The census of 1870 counted 7.1 million horses and 1.1 million mules, as well as 39 million humans. With most urban horses and mules incapacitated for a week or two, humans used wheelbarrows and pulled the wagons. About 1% of the animals died, and the rest fully recovered.

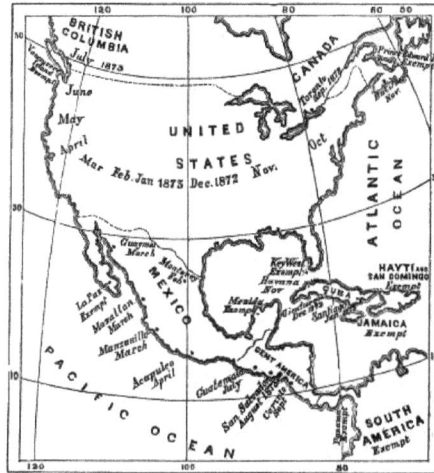

MAP OF NORTH AMERICA, SHOWING THE COURSE OF THE EPIZOÖTIC OF 1872-73.

Spread of epizootic

The first cases of the disease were reported from Ontario, Canada. By October 1, 1872, the first case occurred in Toronto. All the street car horses and major livery stables were affected within only three days. By the middle of October, the disease had reached Montreal, Detroit, and New England. On October 25, 1872, *The New York Times* reported on the extent of the outbreak, claiming that nearly all publistables in the city had been affected, and that the majority of the horses owned in the private sector had essentially been rendered useless to their owners. Only days later, the *Times* went on to report that 95% of all horses in Rochester, New York, had been affected, while the disease was also making its way quickly through the state of Maine and had already affected all fire horses in the city of Providence, Rhode Island.

On October 30, 1872, *The New York Times* reported that a complete suspension of travel had been noted in the state. The same report also took note of massive freight backups being caused by the lack of transportation ability that was arising as a result of the outbreak. Cities such as Buffalo and New York were left without effective ways to move merchandise through the streets, and even the Erie Canal was left with boats full of goods idling in its waters because they were pulled by horses. By November, many states were reporting cases. The street railway industry ground to a halt in late 1872.

Boston was hard hit by a major fire downtown on November 9 as firemen pulled the necessary firefighting equipment by hand. The city commission investigating the fire found that fire crews' response times were delayed by only a matter of minutes. The city then began to buy steam-powered equipment.

In New York, 7,000 of the city's approximately 11,000 horses fell ill, and mortality rates ranged between 1.0% and 10%. Many horses were unable to stand in their stalls. Those that could stand coughed violently and were too weak to pull any loads or support riders. The vast majority of affected horses – save for those 10% that died as a result – were back to full health by the following spring.

2007 Australian Outbreak

Australia had remained free of equine influenza until an outbreak in August 2007. While the virus was successfully contained and Australia has returned to its equine influenza-free status, the outbreak had significant effects on the country's horse-racing industry.

Prevention

Prevention of equine influenza outbreaks is maintained through vaccines and hygiene procedures. Countries that are equine influenza-free normally impose strict and rigorous quarantine measures.

Vaccines

Vaccines (ATCvet codes: QI05AA01 (WHO) inactivated, QI05AD02 (WHO) live, plus various combinations) are a major defense against the disease. Vaccination schedules generally require a primary course of vaccines, followed by booster shots. Standard schedules may not maintain absolutely foolproof levels of protection, and more frequent administration is advised in high-risk situations.

Equine influenza virus (EIV) undergoes continuous antigenidrift, and vaccine protection from immunogenistimulation is maximised when vaccines strains have greater homogeneity to circulating strains. Subclinically affected vaccinated horses can shed live virus and represent a threat to unvaccinated or inappropriately vaccinated horses. Neutralising immunity leading to an absence of infection is rare. (Paillot, 2014). An OIE expert surveillance panel annually assesses circulating strains and makes relevant vaccine recommendations.

The UK requires horses participating in show events be vaccinated against equine flu, and a vaccination card must be produced; the International Federation for Equestrian Sports requires vaccination every six months.

Chronic Wasting Disease

Chroniwasting disease (CWD) is a transmissible spongiform encephalopathy (TSE) of mule deer, white-tailed deer, elk (or "wapiti"), and moose ("elk" in Europe). As of 2016,

CWD had only been found in members of the deer family. First recognized as a clinical "wasting" syndrome in 1967 in mule deer in a wildlife research facility in northern Colorado, USA, it was identified as a TSE in 1978 and has spread to free-ranging and captive populations in 23 US states and two Canadian provinces. CWD is typified by chroniweight loss leading to death. No relationship is known between CWD and any other TSE of animals or people.

Although reports in the popular press have been made of humans being affected by CWD, a study by the Centers for Disease Control and Prevention suggests, "[m]ore epidemiologiand laboratory studies are needed to monitor the possibility of such transmissions." The epidemiological study further concluded, "[a]s a precaution, hunters should avoid eating deer and elk tissues known to harbor the CWD agent (e.g., brain, spinal cord, eyes, spleen, tonsils, lymph nodes) from areas where CWD has been identified."

Clinical Signs

Most cases of CWD occur in adult animals; the youngest animal diagnosed with natural CWD was 17 months. The disease is progressive and always fatal. The first signs are difficulties in movement. The most obvious and consistent clinical sign of CWD is weight loss over time. Behavioral changes also occur in the majority of cases, including decreased interactions with other animals, listlessness, lowering of the head, tremors, repetitive walking in set patterns, and nervousness. Excessive salivation and grinding of the teeth also are observed. Most deer show increased drinking and urination; the increased drinking and salivation may contribute to the spread of the disease.

Causative Agent

The agent responsible for CWD (and other TSEs, such as scrapie and bovine spongiform encephalopathy) is PRNP which is highly conserved among mammals and has been found and sequenced in deer. It is a prion, an abnormal form of a normal protein, known as prion protein (PrP), most commonly found in the central nervous system (CNS), and is capable of spreading to the peripheral nervous system (PNS), thus infecting meat, or muscle, of deer and elk. The abnormal PrP infects the host animal by promoting conversion of normal cellular prion protein (PrP^C) to the abnormal prion form (PrP^{res} or PrP^d). The build-up of PrP^d in the brain is associated with widespread neurodegeneration.

Diagnosis

Diagnosis is based on *post mortem* examination (necropsy) and testing; examination of the dead body is not definitive as many animals die early in the course of the disease and conditions found are non-specific; general signs of poor health and Aspiration pneumonia, which may be the actual cause of death, are common. On microscopiexamination, lesions of CWD in the central nervous system resemble those of other TSEs. In addition, scientists use immunohistochemistry to test brain, lymph, and neuroendocrine tissues for the presence of the abnormal prion protein to diagnose CWD; positive IHfindings in the obex is considered the gold standard.

As of 2015 there were no commercially feasible diagnostitests that could be used on live animals. It is possible to run a bioassay, taking fluids from cervids suspected of infection and incubating them in transgenimice that express the cervid prion protein, to determine if the cervid is infected, but there are ethical issues with this and it is not scalable.

Epidemiology

The origin and mode of transmission of the prions causing CWD is unknown, but recent research indicates that prions can be excreted by deer and elk, and are transmitted by eating grass growing in contaminated soil. Animals born in captivity and those born in the wild have been affected with the disease. Based on epidemiology, transmission of CWD is thought to be lateral (from animal to animal). Maternal transmission may occur, although it appears to be relatively unimportant in maintaining epidemics. An infected deer's saliva is able to spread the CWD prions.

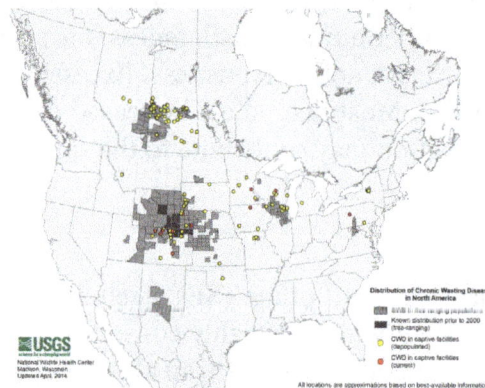

Chroniwasting disease in North America

The disease was first identified in 1967 in a closed herd of captive mule deer in contiguous portions of northeastern Colorado. In 1980, the disease was determined to be a TSE. It was first identified in wild elk and mules in 1981 in Colorado and Wyoming, and in farmed elk in 1997.

In May 2001, CWD was also found in free-ranging deer in the southwestern corner of Nebraska (adjacent to Colorado and Wyoming) and later in additional areas in western Nebraska. The limited area of northern Colorado, southern Wyoming, and western Nebraska in which free-ranging deer, moose, and/or elk positive for CWD have been found is referred to as the endemiarea. The area in 2006 has expanded to six states, including parts of eastern Utah, southwestern South Dakota, and northwestern Kansas.

Also, areas not contiguous (to the endemiarea) areas in central Utah and central Nebraska have been found. The limits of the affected areas are not well defined, since the disease is at a low incidence and the amount of sampling may not be adequate to detect it. In 2002, CWD was detected in wild deer in south-central Wisconsin and northern Illinois and in an isolated area of southern New Mexico. In 2005, it was found in wild white-tailed deer in New York and in Hampshire County, West Virginia. In 2008, the first confirmed case of CWD in Michigan was discovered in an infected deer on an enclosed deer-breeding facility. It is also found in the Canadian provinces of Alberta and Saskatchewan.

In February 2011, the Maryland Department of Natural Resources reported the first confirmed case of the disease in that state. The affected animal was a white-tailed deer killed by a hunter.

CWD has also been diagnosed in farmed elk and deer herds in a number of states and in two Canadian provinces. The first positive farmed elk herd in the United States was detected in 1997 in South Dakota. Since then, additional positive elk herds and farmed white-tailed deer herds have been found in South Dakota (7), Nebraska (4), Colorado (10), Oklahoma (1), Kansas (1), Minnesota (3), Montana (1), Wisconsin (6) and New York (2). As of fall of 2006, four positive elk herds in Colorado and a positive white-tailed deer herd in Wisconsin remain under state quarantine. All of the other herds have been depopulated or have been slaughtered and tested, and the quarantine has been lifted from one herd that underwent rigorous surveillance with no further evidence of disease. CWD also has been found in farmed elk in the Canadian provinces of Saskatchewan and Alberta. A retrospective study also showed mule deer exported from Denver to the Toronto Zoo in the 1980s were affected. In June 2015, the disease was detected in a male white-tailed deer on a breeding ranch in Medina County, Texas. State officials euthanized 34 deer in an effort to contain a possible outbreak.

Species that have been affected with CWD include elk, mule deer, white-tailed deer, black-tailed deer, and moose. Other ruminant species, including wild ruminants and domesticcattle, sheep, and goats, have been housed in wildlife facilities in direct or indirect contact with CWD-affected deer and elk, with no evidence of disease transmission. However, experimental transmission of CWD into other ruminants by intracranial inoculation does result in disease, suggesting only a weak molecular species barrier exists. Research is ongoing to further explore the possibility of transmission of CWD to other species.

By April 2016 CWD had been found in captive animals in South Korea; the disease arrived there with live elk that were imported for farming in the late 1990s.

Europe

In March 2016, a case of CWD was identified in a wild reindeer in Sogn og Fjordane county, Norway. In each of May and June, infected wild moose were found around 300 km north from the first case, in Selbu. By the end of August, a fourth case had been confirmed in a wild reindeer shot in the same area as the first case in March.

Transmission Pathways

Direct Transmission

CWD may be directly transmitted via contact with infected animals, their bodily tissues, and their bodily fluids. Transmission may result from contact with both clinically affected and infected, but asymptomatic, cervids.

Recent research on Rocky Mountain elk found that with CWD-infected dams, many sub-clinical, there was a high rate (80%) of maternal-to-offspring transmission of CWD prions, regardless of gestational period. While not dispositive relative to disease development in the fetus, this does suggest that maternal transmission may be yet another important route of direct CWD transmission.

Experimental Transmission

In addition to the cervid species in which CWD is known to naturally occur, Black-tailed deer and European red deer have been clinically demonstrated to be naturally susceptible to CWD. Other cervid species, including reindeer and caribou, are also suspected to be naturally vulnerable to this disease. Many other non-cervid mammalian species have been experimentally infected with CWD, either orally or via intracerebral inoculation. These species include monkeys, sheep, cattle, prairie voles, mice, and ferrets.

Indirect/Environmental Transmission

Environmental transmission has been linked to contact with infected bodily fluids and tissues, as well as contact with contaminated environments. Once in the environment, CWD prions may remain infectious for many years. Thus, decomposition of diseased carcasses, infected "gut piles" from hunters who field dress their cervid harvests, as well as the urine, saliva, feces, and antler velvet of infected individuals that are deposited in the environment, all have the potential to create infectious environmental reservoirs of CWD.

One avian scavenger, the American crow, was recently evaluated as a potential vector for CWD. As CWD prions remain viable after passing through the bird's digestive tract, crows represent a possible mechanism for the creation of environmental reservoirs of CWD. Additionally, the crows' extensive geographirange presents ample opportunities for them to come in contact with CWD. This coupled with the population density and longevity of communal roosting sites in both urban and rural locations suggests that the fecal deposits at roosting sites may represent a CWD environmental reservoir. Conservative estimates for crows' fecal deposits at *one* winter roosting site for *one* winter season ranged from 391,552 - 599,032 kg.

CWD prions adhere to tightly to soil surface particles and the ground itself becomes a source of infection and may be a major route of transmission due to frequent ground contact when cervids graze.

The Potential for Human Exposure to CWD

As of 2013 there was no evidence of transmission to humans from cervids, nor by eating cervids, but both channels remain a subject of publihealth surveillance and research.

Research

Research is focused on better ways to monitor disease in the wild, live animal diagnostitests, developing vaccines, better ways to dispose of animals who died from the disease and to decontaminate the environment, where prions can persist in soils, and better ways to monitor the food supply.

Parvovirus

Parvovirus is the common name applied to all the viruses in the *Parvoviridae* taxonomifamily. The *Parvoviridae* family has two subfamilies; the *Parvovirinae* (vertebrate viruses) and the *Densovirinae* (invertebrate viruses). Different examples can be given for the subfamily Parvovirinae but the most common is *Dependovirus*, which only work with a helper virus such as adenovirus. Other viruses that can infect without helper viruses are called as autonomous parvoviruses.

Parvoviruses are linear, non-segmented single-stranded DNA viruses, with an average genome size of 5000 nucleotides. They are classified as group II viruses in the Baltimore classification of viruses. Parvoviruses are among the smallest viruses (hence the name, from Latin *parvus* meaning *small*) and are 18–28 nm in diameter.

Parvoviruses can cause disease in some animals, including starfish and humans. Because the viruses require actively dividing cells to replicate, the type of tissue infected varies with the age of the animal. The gastrointestinal tract and lymphatisystem can be affected at any age, leading to vomiting, diarrhea and immunosuppression but cerebellar hypoplasia is only seen in cats that were infected in the womb or at less than two weeks of age, and disease of the myocardium is seen in puppies infected between the ages of three and eight weeks.

History

Perhaps due to their extremely small size, parvoviruses were only recently discovered. Dependoviruses, the first parvoviruses to be discovered, were first isolated in the 1960s. Parvovirus B19, the first known parvovirus to infect humans, was discovered in London by Australian virologist Yvonne Cossart in 1974. Cossart and her group were focused on hepatitis B and were processing blood samples when they discovered a number of "false positives" later identified as parvovirus B19. The virus is named for the patient code of one of the blood bank samples involved in the discovery.

Structure

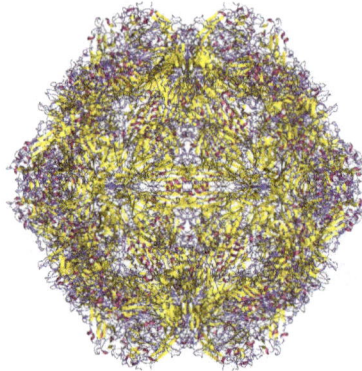

Parvovirus coat protein homo60mer, Carnivore protoparvovirus 1.

The viral capsid of a parvovirus is made up of two to four proteins, known as VP1-4 that form an icosahedral symmetry that is resistant to acids, bases, solvents and temperature up to 50 °(122 degrees Fahrenheit). The capsid is also constructed from 60 protein molecules and one of them creates the majority of the viral capsid structure. Parvoviruses do not have envelopes and are thus considered "naked" viruses. In addition, the shape of the virion is roughly spherical, with surface protrusions and canyons.

Inside the capsid is a linear single-stranded DNA genome in the size range 4–6 kb so the small genome of parvovirus can encode only a few proteins. At the 5' and 3' ends of this genome are short complementary sequences of approximately 120 to 250 nucleotides, that form secondary structures as hairpins for example inverted terminal repeats (ITRs which are two identical secondary structures at the termini) or unique sequences at the termini (there are two unique and different secondary structures at each end of the DNA) and are essential for viral genome replication mechanism called rolling-hairpin replication.

Examples of Parvoviruses

Dependoviruses

Dependoviruses require helper viruses (e.g. herpesviruses) to replicate. They are also perfect candidates as gene vectors. They are utilized to investigate genes in cell cultures of the proteins which are encoded by those genes via mass production method or manipulated as probable vectors to examine genes in the cells of patients for diagnosis and treatment of several genetidiseases and cancers. The biggest advantage for such applications is that they are not known to cause any diseases.

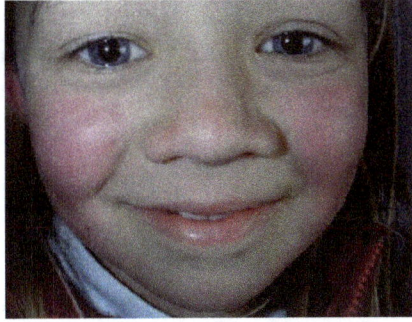

Child with fifth disease.

Autonomous Parvoviruses

Autonomous Parvoviruses do not require a helper virus like dependoviruses. The virus B19 was discovered in blood serum and infects red blood cell precursors. Some infections do not result in visible infection, while some manifest with visible effects, such as fifth disease (erythema infectiosum), which can give children a 'slapped-cheek' appearance.

Disease Information on Parvoviridae

The remainder of this section discusses the disease-causing *Parvoviridae*.

Diseases Caused by Members of the Parvoviridae Family

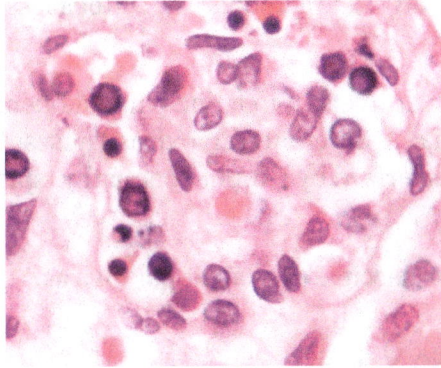

Micrograph showing parvovirus infected nucleated (fetal) red blood cells. H&E stain.

Parvovirus B19, which causes fifth disease in humans, is a member of the *Erythrovirus* genus of the *Parvoviridae*.

Prior to 2014, it was also the name applied to a genus within the subfamily *Parvovirinae*, but this has been amended to genus *Protoparvovirus* to avoid confusion between taxonomilevels. Parvoviruses that infect vertebrate hosts make up the subfamily *Parvovirinae*, while those that infect arthropods (currently only known to infect insects or shrimp) make up the subfamily *Densovirinae*.

Many mammalian species sustain infection by multiple parvoviruses. Parvoviruses tend to be specifiabout the species of animal they will infect, but this is a somewhat flexible characteristic. Thus, all isolates of canine parvovirus affect dogs, wolves, and foxes, but only some of them will infect cats.

Humans can be infected by viruses from five of the eight genera in the subfamily *Parvovirinae*: i) *Bocaparvovirus* (e.g. human bocavirus 1), ii) *Dependoparvovirus* (e.g. adeno-associated virus 2), iii) *Erythroparvovirus* (e.g. parvovirus B19), iv) *Protoparvovirus* (e.g. bufavirus 1a) and v) *Tetraparvovirus* (e.g. human parv4 G1). As of 2014, there were no known human viruses in the remaining three recognized genera: vi) *Amdoparvovirus* (e.g. Aleutian mink disease virus), vii) *Aveparvovirus* (e.g. chicken parvovirus) and viii) *Copiparvovirus* (e.g. bovine parvovirus 2).

Canine parvovirus is a particularly deadly disease among young puppies, about 80% fatal, causing gastrointestinal tract damage and dehydration as well as a cardiasyndrome in very young animals. It is spread by contact with an infected dog's feces. Symptoms include lethargy, severe diarrhea, fever, vomiting, loss of appetite, and dehydration.

Mouse parvovirus 1, however, causes no symptoms but can contaminate immunology experiments in biological research laboratories.

Porcine parvovirus causes a reproductive disease in swine known as SMEDI, which stands for stillbirth, mummification, embryonideath, and infertility.

Feline panleukopenia is common in kittens and causes fever, low white blood cell count, diarrhea, and death. Infection of the cat fetus and kittens less than two weeks old causes cerebellar hypoplasia.

Mink enteritis virus is similar in effect to feline panleukopenia, except that it does not cause cerebellar hypoplasia. A different parvovirus causes Aleutian Disease in mink and other mustelids, characterized by lymphadenopathy, splenomegaly, glomerulonephritis, anemia, and death.

Dogs, cats and swine can be vaccinated against parvovirus.

Replication as Disease Vector

To enter host cells, parvoviruses bind to a sialiacid-bearing cell surface receptor. Penetration into the cytoplasm is mediated by a phospholipase A2 activity carried on the amino-terminal peptide of the capsid VP1 polypeptide. Once in the cytoplasm, the intact virus is translocated to the nucleus prior to uncoating. Transcription only initiates when the host cell enters S-phase under its own cell cycle control, at which time the cell's replication machinery converts the incoming single strand into a duplex transcription template, allowing synthesis of mRNAs encoding the non-structural proteins, NS1 and NS2. The mRNAs are transported out of the nucleus into the cytoplasm where the host ribosomes translate them into viral proteins. Viral DNA replication proceeds through a series of monomeriand concatemeriduplex intermediates by a unidirectional strand-displacement mechanism that is mediated by components of the host replication fork, aided and orchestrated by the viral NS1 polypeptide. NS1 also transactivates an internal transcriptional promoter that directs synthesis of the structural VP polypeptides. Once assembled capsids are available, replication shifts from synthesizing duplex DNA to displacement of progeny single strands, which are typically negative-sense and are packaged in a 3'-to-5' direction into preformed particles within the nucleus. Mature virions may be released from infected cells prior to cell lysis, which promotes rapid transmission of the virus, but if this fails then the virus is released at cell lysis.

Unlike most other DNA viruses, parvoviruses are unable to activate DNA synthesis in host cells. Thus, in order for viral replication to take place the infected cells must be non-quiescent (i.e. must be actively mitotic). Their inability to force host cells into S-phase means that parvoviruses are non-tumorigenic. Indeed, they are commonly oncolytic, showing a strong tendency to replicate preferentially in cells with transformed phenotypes.

Use of HeLa Cells in Parvovirus Testing

Testing for how feline parvovirus and canine parvovirus infect cells and what pathways are taken; scientists used cat cells, mouse cells, cat and mouse hybrid cells, mink cells, dog cells, human cells, and HeLa cells. Both feline parvovirus and canine parvovirus enter their hosts, follow specifipathways, and infect at certain parts of cells before infecting major organs. Parvoviruses are specifiviruses that are characterized by which receptors they attack. Testing found that parvovirus infects carnivorous animals through the oropharyngeal pathway. Parvovirus infects the oropharyngeal cells that come in immediate contact with the virus. It contains a plasmid that infects and binds to transferrin receptors, a glycoprotein, on the plasma membrane. The parvovirus plasmid is stored in a small non-enveloped capsid. Once oropharyngeal cells become infected the virus spreads to dividing lymph cells and continues to work to the bone marrow and spread to target organs through blood.

Testing of HeLa cells and human cells to exposure of both feline parvovirus and canine parvovirus resulted in infections of the cells at human transferrin receptors. When antibodies and parvovirus samples were added at the same time to human cells and HeLa cells it was found that no infection would take place; experiments showed that both human cells and HeLa cells have transferrin receptors but there is no evidence of humans contracting parvovirus.

Certain chromosomes in cells show more susceptibility to parvovirus than others. Testing of feline parvovirus on cat cells and cat mouse hybrid cells found cultures with cells having the highest concentrations of the C2 chromosome were the most highly infected cells. Slight mutations of binding sites were found to slow down or completely stop the infection of the given parvovirus; whereas cells that are naturally missing the receptors or are mutants lacking them cannot be mutated. Both feline parvovirus and canine parvovirus express plasticity during cellular infection. Although transferrin receptors may be limited on cell surfaces the parvovirus will find available transferrin receptors and will use different pathways to gain entry to the cell. Unlike plasma membrane infection plasticity, all strains of parvovirus show related routes to the cell nucleus.

Canine and Feline

Canine parvovirus is a mutant strain of feline parvovirus. A very specifimutation is necessary for the virus to change species of infection. The mutation affects capsid proteins of feline parvovirus giving it the ability to infect dogs. Both forms of the virus are very similar, so once the mutation has occurred, canine parvovirus is still able to infect cats. The canine parvovirus has the tradeoff of gaining the ability to infect canine cells while becoming less effective at infecting feline cells. Both feline parvovirus and canine parvovirus bind to and infect the transferrin receptors, but both have different sequences in the cells and animals. Infection by both feline parvovirus and canine parvovirus are relatively quick; but because of constant mutation of canine parvovirus, canine parvovirus has a slower infection time than feline parvovirus. Studies of other strains of mutated canine parvovirus have revealed that changes in the viral capsid by just one protein can be fatal to the virus. Deleterious mutations have been noted to lead to inability to bind to transferrin receptors, bind to non- receptive parts of the cell membrane, and identification of the virus by the host's antibody cells.

Management and Therapy

Currently there is no vaccine to prevent infection by parvoviruses, but recently the virus's capsid proteins, which are noninfectious molecules, have been suggested acting as antigens for improving of vaccines.

Antivirals and human immunoglobulin sourced treatments are usually for relief of symptoms. Utilizing immunoglobulins is a logical solution for treatment as neutralizing antibodies because a majority of adults have been in danger from the parvoviruses especially B19 virus.

Canine Transmissible Venereal Tumor

Canine transmissible venereal tumors (CTVTs), also called transmissible venereal tumors (TVTs), canine transmissible venereal sarcoma (CTVS), sticker tumors and infectious sarcoma is a histiocytitumor of the external genitalia of the dog and other canines, and is transmitted from animal to animal during mating. It is one of only four known transmissible cancers; another is devil facial tumor disease, a cancer which occurs in Tasmanian devils.

The tumor cells are themselves the infectious agents, and the tumors that form are not genetically related to the host dog. Although the genome of a CTVT is derived from a canid (probably a dog, wolf or coyote), it is now essentially living as a unicellular, asexually reproducing (but sexually transmitted) pathogen. Sequence analysis of the genome suggests it diverged from canids over 6,000 years ago; possibly much earlier. The most recent estimates of its time of origin place date it to about 11,000 years ago. However, the most recent common ancestor of *extant* tumors is more recent: it probably originated 200 to 2,500 years ago.

Canine TVTs were initially described by Russian veterinarian M.A. Novinsky (1841–1914) in 1876, when he demonstrated that the tumor could be transplanted from one dog to another by infecting them with tumor cells.

Biology

Canine transmissible venereal tumors are histiocytitumors that may be transmitted among dogs through coitus, licking, biting and sniffing tumor affected areas. The concept that the tumor is naturally transmissible as an allograft came from three important observations. First, CTVTs can only be experimentally induced by transplanting living tumor cells, and not by killed cells or cell filtrates. Second, the tumor karyotype is aneuploid but has characteristimarker chromosomes in all tumors collected in different geographiregions. Third, a long interspersed nuclear element (LINE-1) insertion near c-myhas been found in all tumors examined so far and can be used as a diagnostimarker to confirm that a tumor is a CTVT.

The CTVT cells have fewer chromosomes than normal cells. Dog cells normally have 78 chromosomes; The cancer cells contain 57–64 chromosomes that are very different in appearance from normal dog chromosomes. All dog chromosomes except X and Y are acrocentric, having a centromere very near to the end of the chromosome, while many of the CTVT chromosomes are metacentrior submetacentric, having a centromere nearer to the middle. There is no evidence that the tumor is caused by a virus or virus-like organism. The infectious agent of canine transmissible venereal tumor is the cancer cell itself and the tumor is clonal in origin. All tumor cells of this type of cancer share extremely similar geneticode, often if not always unrelated to the DNA of their host. Specifically, the LINE-1 element in the tumor cells is in a different location than in normal canine DNA. This demonstrates that the tumors do not arise from separate cancerous transformation in individual animals. Rather, the malignant tumor cells from one dog are transferred to another.

Canine transmissible venereal tumors are most commonly seen in sexually active dogs in tropical and subtropical climates. The disease is spread when dogs mate, and it can even be transmitted to other canine species, such as foxes and coyotes. Spontaneous regression of the tumor can occur, probably due to a response from the immune system. CTVT undergoes a predictable cycle: the initial growth phase of four to six months (P phase), a stable phase, and a regression phase (R phase), although not all CTVTs will regress. The tumor does not often metastasize (occurring in about 5 percent of cases), except in puppies and immunocompromised dogs. Metastasis is most commonly to regional lymph nodes, but can also be seen in the skin, brain, eye, liver, spleen, testicle, and muscle. A biopsy is necessary for diagnosis.

The success of this single cell lineage, believed to be the longest continually propagated cell lineage in the world, can be attributed to the tumor's mode of transmission in a specifihost system. Although direct contact is generally not a highly efficient mode of transfer, CTVTs take advantage of the popular sire effect of domestidogs. A single male can produce dozens of litters over his lifetime, allowing the tumor to affect many more females than it could if a monogamous species were the host. Understanding the epidemiology of CTVTs is hoped to provide insights for populations that may experience CTVT exposure and information about disease prevalence. Canine transmissible venereal tumors are more often found in temperate climates where there are large populations of stray dogs, but little is known about the details of transmission.

Signs and Symptoms

In male dogs, the tumor affects the penis and foreskin. In female dogs, it affects the vulva. Rarely, the mouth or nose are affected. The tumor often has a cauliflower-like appearance. Signs of genital TVT include a discharge from the prepuce and in some cases urinary retention, from blockage of the urethra. Signs of a nasal TVT include nasal fistulae, nosebleeds and other nasal discharge, facial swelling, and enlargement of the submandibular lymph nodes.

Treatment

Surgery may be difficult due to the location of these tumors. Surgery alone often leads to recurrence. Chemotherapy is very effective for TVTs. The prognosis for complete remission with chemotherapy is excellent. The most common chemotherapy agents used are vincristine, vinblastine, and doxorubicin. Radiotherapy may be required if chemotherapy does not work.

Devil Facial Tumour Disease

Devil facial tumour disease (DFTD) is an aggressive non-viral transmissible parasiticancer among Tasmanian devils.

The first official case of DFTD was described in 1996 in Australia. In the subsequent decade the disease ravaged Tasmania's wild devils, with estimates of decline ranging from 20% to as much as 50% of the devil population, across over 65% of the state. Affected high-density populations suffer up to 100% mortality in 12–18 months. The disease has mainly been concentrated in Tasmania's eastern half. Visible signs of DFTD begin with lesions and lumps around the mouth. These develop into cancerous tumours that may spread from the face to the entire body. Devils usually die within six months from organ failure, secondary infection, or metabolistarvation as the tumours interfere with feeding. DFTD affects males and females equally. At present the population has dwindled by 70% since 1996. As of 2010, 80% of population is infected.

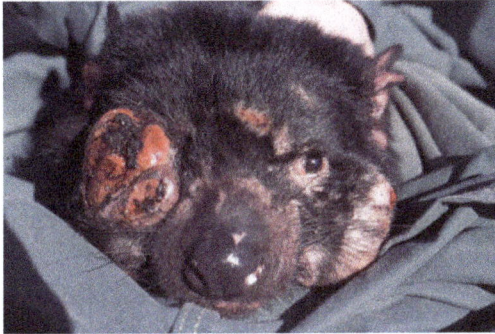

Devil facial tumour disease causes tumours to form in and around the mouth, interfering with feeding and eventually leading to death by starvation.

The most plausible route of transmission is through biting, particularly when canine teeth come into direct contact with the diseased cells. Other modes of transmission include the ingesting of an infected carcass and the sharing of food, both of which involve an allogeneitransfer of cells between unrelated individuals.

Six females have been found with a partial immunity. Breeding in captivity has begun in an attempt to save the population.

Characteristics

Tasmanian devil cells have 14 chromosomes, while the oldest-known strain of the tumour cell contains thirteen chromosomes, nine of which are recognizable and four of which are mutated "marker" chromosomes. More recently evolved strains have an additional mutant marker chromosome, for a total of fourteen chromosomes. Researchers identified the cancer as a neuroendocrine tumour, and found identical chromosomal rearrangements in all the cancer cells. The karyotype anomalies of DFTD cells are similar to those of cancer cells from canine transmissible venereal tumour (CTVT), a cancer of dogs that is transmitted by physical contact. Among the different alterations present in the tumour genome can be found several single base mutations or shorts insertions and deletions (indels) like deletions in the chromosomes 1, 2 and 3, as well as trisomy in 5p. Some of the mutated or deleted genes in DFTD are RET, FANCD2, MAST3 and BTNL9-like gene.

The theory that cancer cells themselves could be an infective agent (the Allograft Theory) was first supported by the researchers A-M. Pearse, K. Swift, and colleagues. In

2006, Pearse and Swift analyzed DFTD cells from several devils in different locations, and determined that all of the DFTD cells were not only genetically identical to each other, but also genetically distinct from their hosts, and from all known Tasmanian devils. Thus the cancer must have originated in a single individual and spread, rather than arising separately within each animal. Twenty one different subtypes have been identified by analyzing the genomes (mitochondrial and nuclear) of 104 tumours from different Tasmanian devils. Later researchers witnessed a previously-uninfected devil develop tumours from lesions caused by an infected devil's bites, confirming that the disease is spread by allograft, and that the normal methods of transmission include biting, scratching, and aggressive sexual activity between individuals. During biting, infection can spread from the bitten devil to the biter. Since June 2005, three females have been found that are partially resistant to DFTD.

Further research from the University of Sydney has shown that the infectious facial cancer may be able to spread because of low diversity in devil immune genes (MHclass I and II). The same genes are also found in the tumours, so the devil's immune system does not recognize the tumour cells as foreign. There are at least four, and most likely more, strains of the cancer, showing that it is evolving, and may become more virulent. Increased levels of tetraploidy have been shown to exist in the oldest strain of DFTD as of 2014, which correlates with the devils involved being subjected to a DFTD removal programme. Because ploidy slows the tumour growth rate, Ujvari et al. posit that the DFTD removal programme selected for slower-growing tumours, and that disease eradication programmes may result in the evolution of DFTD. The strains may also complicate attempts to develop a vaccine, and the mutation of the cancer may mean that it could spread to other related species, like the quoll.

In a paper published in the January 2010 issue of *Science*, an international team of researchers announced that devil facial tumour disease likely originated in the Schwann cells of a single devil. Schwann cells are found in the peripheral nervous system, and produce myelin and other proteins essential for the functions of nerve cells in the peripheral nervous system. The researchers sampled 25 tumours and found that the tumours were genetically identical. Using deep sequencing technology, they then profiled the tumours' transcriptome, the set of genes that are active in tumours. The transcriptomes closely matched those of Schwann cells, revealing high activity in many of the genes coding for myelin basiprotein production. Several specifimarkers were identified by the team, including the MBP and PRX genes, which may enable veterinarians to more easily distinguish DFTD from other types of cancer, and may eventually help identify a genetipathway that can be targeted to treat it.

Due to the decreased life expectancy of the devils due to DFTD, they have begun breeding at younger ages in the wild, with reports that many only live to participate in one breeding cycle. A study has suggested that Tasmanian devils have changed their breeding habits in response to the disease. Females previously started breeding at the age of two, then annually for about three more years until dying normally. Now they commonly breed at the age of one, and die of tumours shortly thereafter. It is speculated that the disease is spread by devils biting each other during the mating season. Social interactions have been seen spreading DFTD in a local area. It is one of three known contagious cancers.

In 2015, a variant form of the cancer was described which was tetraploid, not diploid like the main form of the cancer. The tetraploid form has been linked to lower mortality rates.

Pathology

Growth of large tumours impedes feeding, and starvation is a common cause of death in affected devils. Organ involvement and additional infections may also be a factor in death, as regional lymph node involvement and systemimetastasis is common. The cancer invades the heart.

The tumours are capable of dissolving parts of the skull.

The tumours are "large, solid, soft tissue masses usually with flattened, centrally ulcerated, and exudative surfaces", which are "typically multicentric, appearing first in the oral, face, or neck regions". The tumours are "circumscribed to infiltrative nodular aggregates of round to spindle-shaped cells, often within a pseudocapsule and divided into lobules by delicate fibrous septae".

Preservation Response

Wild Tasmanian devil populations are being monitored to track the spread of the disease and to identify changes in disease prevalence. Field monitoring involves trapping devils within a defined area to check for the presence of the disease and determine the number of affected animals. The same area is visited repeatedly to characterise the spread of the disease over time. So far, it has been established that the short-term effects of the disease in an area can be severe. Long-term monitoring at replicated sites will be essential to assess whether these effects remain, or whether populations can recover. Field workers are also testing the effectiveness of disease suppression by trapping and removing diseased devils. It is hoped that the removal of diseased devils from wild populations should decrease disease prevalence and allow more devils to survive beyond their juvenile years and breed. A study felt that the current system of culling did not impede the disease's spread.

Two "insurance" populations of disease-free devils are being established at an urban facility in the Hobart suburb of Taroona and on Maria Island off the east coast of Tasmania. Captive breeding in mainland zoos is also a possibility. The decline in devil numbers is also seen as an ecological problem, since its presence in the Tasmanian forest ecosystem is believed to have prevented the establishment of the red fox, illegally introduced to Tasmania in 2001. It is believed that Tasmanian devil young would be vulnerable to red fox predation, as they are left alone for long periods of time.

In response to the impact of DFTD on Tasmanian devil populations, 47 devils have been shipped to mainland Australian wildlife parks to attempt to preserve the genetidiversity of the species. The largest of these efforts is the Devil Ark project in Barrington Tops, New South Wales; an initiative of the Australian Reptile Park. This project aims to create a set of one thousand genetically representative devils, and is now a major focus of the insurance policy. In addition, the Tasman peninsula is being considered as a possible "clean area" with the single narrow access point controlled by physical barriers. The Tasmanian Department of Primary Industries and Water is experimenting on culling infected animals with some signs of success.

In 2008, a devil named Cedriwas thought to have a natural immunity to the disease, but in late 2008 he developed two tumours on his face. The tumours were removed and officials thought Cedriwas responding well until September 2010 when it was discovered that the cancer had spread to his lungs. He was euthanized upon the discovery. A diagnostiblood test was developed in mid-2009 to screen for the disease. In early 2010, scientists found some Tasmanian devils, mostly in the north-west of Tasmania, that are genetically different enough for their bodies to recognise the cancer as foreign. They have only one Major Histocompatibility Complex, whereas the cancerous cells have both.

At present with the population reduced by 70% since 1996, if a cure is not found then scientists predict they will become extinct by 2035.

A study recommended oocyte banking be used in the conservation effort for Tasmanian devils, as the survival rate of the oocytes in their study was 70%.

In 2010, there was hope that EBC-46, a drug which cures facial tumours in dogs, cats, and horses, may be a cure for DFTD.

Vaccination with irradiated cancer cells has not proven successful.

Research published in the *Proceedings of the National Academy of Sciences* on June 27, 2011, suggests picking a genetically diverse breeding stock, defined by the genome sequence, for conservation efforts.

In 2011, Principal Investigator David Phalen, (Wildlife Health and Conservation Centre, University of Sydney) and Stephen Pyecroft (Department of Primary Industries and Water in Tasmania) along with Antony Moore and Angela Frimberger (Veterinary Oncology Consultants) were awarded a Tasmanian Government Project Management Grant for their project Investigation into Chemotherapy Agents Effective Against the Tasmanian Devil Facial Tumour.

In 2013, a study using mice as a model for Tasmanian devils suggested that a DFTD vaccine or treatment could be beneficial.

In 2015, a study which mixed dead DFTD cells with an inflammatory substance caused an immune response in five out of six devils injected with the mixture. This has created hopes for a vaccine against DFTD. Field testing of the potential vaccine is being undertaken as a collaborative project between the Menzies Institute for Medical Research and the Save the Tasmanian Devil Program under the Wild Devil Recovery program, and aims to test the immunisation protocol as a tool in ensuring the devil's long term survival in the wild.

History

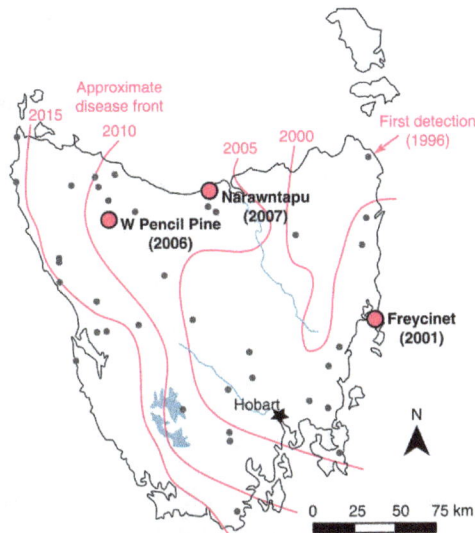

Spread of the disease as of 2015

In 1996, a photographer from The Netherlands captured several images of devils with facial tumours near Mount William in Tasmania's northeast. Around the same time, farmers reported a decline in devil numbers. Menna Jones first encountered the disease in 1999 near Little Swanport, in 2001 capturing three devils with facial tumours on the Freycinet Peninsula.

The devil population on the peninsula decreased dramatically. In March 2003 Nick Mooney wrote a memo to be circulated within the Parks and Wildlife Services calling for more funding to study the disease, but the call for funding was edited out before the memo was presented to Bryan Green, then Tasmania's Minister for Primary Industries, Water and Environment. In April 2003, a working group was formed by the Tasmanian Government to respond to the disease. In September 2003, Nick Mooney went to the Tasmanian daily newspaper *The Mercury*, informing the general publiof the disease and proposing a quarantine of healthy Tasmanian devils. At the time, it was thought that a retrovirus was a possible cause. David Chadwick of the state Animal Health Laboratory said that the laboratory did not have the resources needed to research the possibility of a retrovirus. The Tasmanian Conservation Trust criticised the Tasmanian government for providing insufficient funds for research and suggested that DFTD could be zoonotic, posing a threat to livestock and humans. On 14 October 2003, a workshop was held in Launceston. In 2004, Kathryn Medlock found three oddly shaped devil skulls in European museums and found a description of a devil in London Zoo dying, which showed a similarity to DFTD.

A virus was initially thought to be the cause of DFTD, but no evidence of such a virus could be detected in the cancer cells. Calicivirus, 1080 poison, agricultural chemicals, and habitat fragmentation combined with a retrovirus were other proposed causes. Environmental toxins had also been suspected. In March 2006 a devil escaped from a park into an area infected with DFTD. She was recaptured with bite marks on her face, and returned to live with the other devils in the park. She wounded a male and by October both devils had DFTD, which was subsequently spread to two others. This incident helped test the viability of the allograft theory of transmission. In 2006, DFTD was classed a List B notifiable disease under the Animal Health Act 1995. Also in 2006, the strategy of developing an insurance population in captivity was developed. It was reassessed in 2008. A 2007 investigation into the immune system of the devils found that when combatting other pathogens, the response from the immune system was normal, leading to suspicion that the devils were not capable of detecting the cancerous cells as "non-self". In 2007, it was predicted that populations could become locally extinct within 10–15 years of DFTD occurring, and predicted that the disease would spread across the entire range of the Tasmanian devils. This study also predicted that Tasmanian devils would become extinct within 25–35 years.

In 2008, high levels of potentially carcinogeniflame retardant chemicals were found in Tasmanian devils. Preliminary results of tests of fat tissue revealed high levels of hexabromobiphenyl (BB153) and "reasonably high" levels of decabromodiphenyl ether (BDE209).

In 2016, devils are at the verge of extinction as the localized populations were shown to be declined by 90 percent and an overall species decline of more than 80 percent in less than 20 years, with some models predicting extinction. Despite this, devil populations persist in disease stricken areas. The devils have, in a way, fought back the extinction by developing the gene that is immune to Face tumors. The genes have already existed in the Tasmanian devil as part of their immune system. They increased in frequency due to natural selection. That is, the individuals with particular forms of these genes (alleles) survived and reproduced disproportionately to those that lacked the specifi- variants when disease was present.

In Other Animals

Transmissible cancer, caused by a clone of malignant cells rather than a virus, is extremely rare, with only two other known transmissible cancers—canine transmissible venereal tumour (CTVT), which is sexually transmitted among dogs, and contagious reticulum cell sarcoma of the Syrian hamster, which can be transmitted via mosquito bites of *Aedes aegypti*. CTVT mutes the expression of the immune response, whereas the Syrian hamster disease spreads due to lack of genetidiversity.

Lymphoma in Animals

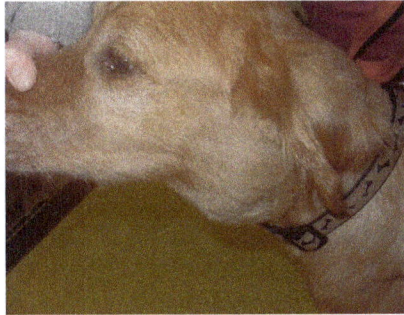

Lymphoma in a Golden Retriever

Lymphoma (lymposarcoma) in animals is a type of cancer defined by a proliferation of malignant lymphocytes within solid organs such as the lymph nodes, bone marrow, liver and spleen. The disease also may occur in the eye, skin, and gastrointestinal tract.

Lymphoma in Dogs

Lymphoma is one of the most common malignant tumors to occur in dogs. The cause is genetic, but there are also suspected environmental factors involved, including in one study an increased risk with the use of the herbicide 2,4-D. This risk was not confirmed in another study.

Breeds that are commonly affected include Boxer, Scottish Terrier, Basset Hound, Airedale Terrier, Chow Chow, German Shepherd, Poodle, St. Bernard, Bulldog, Beagle, Rottweiler and Golden Retriever. The Golden Retriever is especially susceptible to developing lymphoma, with a lifetime risk of 1:8.

Classification

The cancer is classified into low and high grade types. Classification is also based on location. The four location types are multicentric, mediastinal, gastrointestinal, and extranodal (involving the kidney, central nervous system, skin, heart, or eye). Multicentrilymphoma, the most common type (by greater than 80 percent), is found in the lymph nodes, with or without involvement in the liver, spleen, or bone marrow. Mediastinal lymphoma occurs in the lymph nodes in the thorax and possibly the thymus. Gastrointestinal lymphoma occurs as either a solitary tumor or diffuse invasion of the stomach or intestines, with or without involvement in the surrounding lymph nodes, liver or spleen. Classification is further based on involvement of B-lymphocytes or T-lymphocytes. Approximately 70 percent are B-cell lymphoma. Cutaneous lymphoma can be classified as epitheliotropi(closely conforming to the epidermis) or non-epitheliotropic. The epitheliotropiform is typically of T-cell origin and is also called mycosis fungoides. The non-epitheliotropiform is typically of B-cell origin.

Signs and Symptoms

General signs and symptoms include depression, fever, weight loss, loss of appetite, loss of hair or fur and vomiting. Lymphoma is the most common cancerous cause of hypercalcemia (high blood calcium levels) in dogs. It can lead to the above signs and symptoms plus increased water drinking, increased urination, and cardiaarrhythmias. Hypercalcemia in these cases is caused by secretion of parathyroid hormone-related protein.

Multicentrilymphoma presents as painless enlargement of the peripheral lymph nodes. This is seen in areas such as under the jaw, the armpits, the groin, and behind the knees. Enlargement of the liver and spleen causes the abdomen to distend. Mediastinal lymphoma can cause fluid to collect around the lungs, leading to coughing and difficulty breathing. Hypercalcemia is most commonly associated with this type.

Gastrointestinal lymphoma causes vomiting, diarrhea, and melena (digested blood in the stool). Low serum albumin levels and hypercalcemia can also occur.

Lymphoma of the skin is an uncommon occurrence. The epitheliotropiform typically appears as itchy inflammation of the skin progressing to nodules and plaques. The non-epitheliotropiform can have a wide variety of appearances, from a single lump to large areas of bruised, ulcerated, hairless skin. The epitheliotropiform must be differentiated from similar appearing conditions such as pemphigus vulgaris, bullous pemphigoid, and lupus erythematosus.

Signs for lymphoma in other sites depend on the location. Central nervous system involvement can cause seizures or paralysis. Eye involvement, seen in 20 to 25 percent of cases, can lead to glaucoma, uveitis, bleeding within the eye, retinal detachment, and blindness. Lymphoma in the bone marrow causes anemia, low platelet count, and low white blood cell count.

Diagnosis

Biopsy of affected lymph nodes or organs confirms the diagnosis, although a needle aspiration of an affected lymph node can increase suspicion of the disease. X-rays, ultrasound and bone marrow biopsy reveal other locations of the cancer. There are now a range of blood tests that can be utilised to aid in the diagnosis of lymphoma. Flow cytometry detects antibodies linked to tumour cell surface antigens in fluid samples or cell suspensions. Polymerase chain reaction (PCR) for antigen receptor rearrangements (PARR) identifies circulating tumour cells based on unique genetisequences. The canine Lymphoma Blood Test (cLBT) measures multiple circulating biomarkers and utilises a complex algorithm to diagnose lymphoma. This test utilises the acute phase proteins (C-Reactive Protein and Haptoglobin). In combination with basiclinical symptoms, it gives in differential diagnosis the sensitivity 83.5% and specificity 77%. The TK canine cancer panel is an indicator of general neoplastidisease. The stage of the disease is important to treatment and prognosis. Certain blood tests have also been shown to be prognostic.

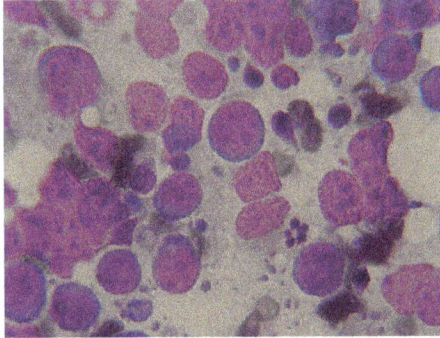

Cytology of lymphoma in a dog

The stage of the disease is important to treatment and prognosis.

- Stage I - only one lymph node or lymphoid tissue in one organ involved.

- Stage II - lymph nodes in only one area of the body involved.

- Stage III - generalized lymph node involvement.

- Stage IV - any of the above with liver or spleen involvement.

- Stage V - any of the above with blood or bone marrow involvement.

Each stage is divided into either *substage a*, those without systemisymptoms; or *substage b*, those with systemisymptoms such as fever, loss of appetite, weight loss, and fatigue.

Treatment

Due to the high risk of recurrence and ensuing problems, close monitoring of dogs undergoing chemotherapy is important. The same is true for dogs that have entered remission and ceased treatment. Monitoring for disease and remission/recurrence is usually performed by palpation of peripheral lymph nodes. This procedure detects gross changes in peripheral lymph nodes. Some of the blood tests used in diagnosing lymphoma also offer greater objectivity and provide an earlier warning of an animal coming out of remission.

Complete cure is rare with lymphoma and treatment tends to be palliative, but long remission times are possible with chemotherapy. With effective protocols, average first remission times are 6 to 8 months. Second remissions are shorter and harder to accomplish. Average survival is 9 to 12 months. The most common treatment is a combination of cyclophosphamide, vincristine, prednisone, L-asparaginase, and doxorubicin. Other chemotherapy drugs such as chlorambucil, lomustine (CCNU), cytosine arabinoside, and mitoxantrone are sometimes used in the treatment of lymphoma by themselves or in substitution for other drugs. In most cases, appropriate treatment protocols cause few side effects, but white blood cell counts must be monitored.

Allogeneiand autologous stem cell transplantations (as is commonly done in humans) have recently been shown to be a possible treatment option for dogs. Most of the basiresearch on transplantation biology was generated in dogs. Current cure rates using stem cell therapy in dogs approximates that achieved in humans, 40-50%.

When cost is a factor, prednisone used alone can improve the symptoms dramatically, but it does not significantly affect the survival rate. The average survival times of dogs treated with prednisone and untreated dogs are both one to two months. Using prednisone alone can cause the cancer to become resistant to other chemotherapy agents, so it should only be used if more aggressive treatment is not an option.

Isotretinoin can be used to treat cutaneous lymphoma.

Prognosis

Untreated dogs have an average survival time of 60 days. Lymphoma with a histologi-high grade generally respond better to treatment but have shorter survival times than dogs with low grade lymphoma. Dogs with B-lymphocyte tumors have a longer survival time than T-lymphocyte tumors. Mediastinal lymphoma has a poorer prognosis than other types, especially those with hypercalcemia. Clinical stage and substage have some prognostivalue, with poorer prognosis associated with Stage V disease, and with substage b (clinical illness at time of presentation).

Lymphoma in Cats

Lymphoma is the most common malignancy diagnosed in cats. Lymphoma in young cats occurs most frequently following infection with feline leukemia virus (FeLV) or to a lesser degree feline immunodeficiency virus (FIV). These cats tend to have involvement of lymph nodes, spine, or mediastinum. Cats with FeLV are 62 times more likely to develop lymphoma, and cats with both FeLV and FIV are 77 times more likely. Younger cats tend to have T-cell lymphoma and older cats tend to have B-cell lymphoma. Older cats tend to have gastrointestinal lymphoma without FeLV infection, although tests more sensitive to low level FeLV infections and replication-defective FeLV have found that many of these cats have been previously exposed. The same forms of lymphoma that are found in dogs also occur in cats, but gastrointestinal is the most common type. Lymphoma of the kidney is the most common kidney tumor in cats, and lymphoma is also the most common heart tumor.

Classification

Gastrointestinal lymphoma is classified into low grade, intermediate grade, and high grade. Low grade types include lymphocytiand small cell lymphoma. High grade types include lymphoblastic, immunoblastic, and large cell lymphoma. Low grade lymphoma is only found in the small intestine, while high grade can commonly be found in the stomach.

Symptoms

Cats that develop lymphoma are much more likely to develop more severe symptoms than dogs. Whereas dogs often appear healthy initially except for swollen lymph nodes, cats will often be physically ill. The symptoms correspond closely to the location of the lymphoma. The most common sites for alimentary (gastrointestinal) lymphoma are, in decreasing frequency, the small intestine, the stomach, the junction of the ileum, cecum, and colon. Cats with the alimentary form of lymphoma often present with weight loss, rough hair coat, loss of appetite, vomiting and diarrhea, although vomiting and diarrhea are commonly absent as symptoms. The tumor can also cause life-threatening blockage of the intestine. Cats with the mediastinal form often have respiratory distress and fluid in the thoracicavity. If lymphoma develops in the kidney, the cat may have increased water consumption and increased urination. Lymphoma of the kidney presents as bilateral kidney enlargement and failure. If the lymphoma is located in the nose, the cat may have discharge from the nose and facial swelling. Lymphoma of the heart causes congestive heart failure, pericardial effusion, and cardiaarrhythmias. Ocular lymphoma in cats often presents as anterior uveitis (inflammation of the inside of the eye). Cats who are also infected with FeLV often present with pale mucous membranes due to anemia. Anemia is a common problem in all cats with lymphoma, but hypercalcemia is rare.

Diagnosis is similar to dogs, except cats should be tested for FeLV and FIV. It is important to differentiate the alimentary form of lymphoma from inflammatory bowel disease because the signs are so similar in cats. A biopsy is necessary to do this. One approach to differentiate inflammatory bowel disease from is to test the infiltrating lymphocytes for their monoclonal origin in lymphomas.

Treatment and Prognosis

Chemotherapy is the mainstay of treatment for lymphoma in cats. Most of the drugs used in dogs are used in cats, but the most common protocol uses cyclophosphamide, vincristine, and prednisone. Gastrointestinal lymphoma has also commonly been treated with a combination of prednisolone and high dose pulse chlorambucil with success. The white blood cell count must be monitored. Remission and survival times are comparable to dogs. Lower stage lymphoma has a better prognosis. Multicentrilymphoma has a better response to treatment than the gastrointestinal form, but infection with FeLV worsens the prognosis.

About 75% of cats treated with chemotherapy for lymphoma go into remission. Unfortunately, after an initial remission, most cats experience a relapse, after which they have a median survival of 6 months. However, about one-third of cats treated with chemotherapy will survive more than 2 years after diagnosis; a small number of these cats may be cured of their disease. Untreated, most cats with lymphoma die within 4–6 weeks. Most cats tolerate their chemotherapy well, and fewer than 5% have severe side effects. Cats do not lose their fur from chemotherapy, though loss of whiskers is possible. Other side effects include low white blood cell count, vomiting, loss of appetite, diarrhea, or fatigue. These can typically be controlled well, and most cats have a good quality of life during treatment. If a cat relapses after attaining remission, the cat can be treated with different chemotherapy drugs to try for a second remission. The chances of a second remission are much lower than the chances of obtaining a first, and the second remission is often shorter than the first.

Lymphoma in Ferrets

Lymphoma is common in ferrets and is the most common cancer in young ferrets. There is some evidence that a retrovirus may play a role in the development of lymphoma like in cats. The most commonly affected tissues are the lymph nodes, spleen, liver, intestine, mediastinum, bone marrow, lung, and kidney.

In young ferrets, the disease progresses rapidly. The most common symptom is difficulty breathing caused by enlargement of the thymus. Other symptoms include loss of appetite, weight loss, weakness, depression, and coughing. It can also masquerade as a chronidisease such as an upper respiratory infection or gastrointestinal disease. In older ferrets, lymphoma is usually chroniand can exhibit no symptoms for years. Symptoms seen are the same as in young ferrets, plus splenomegaly, abdominal masses, and peripheral lymph node enlargement.

Diagnosis is through biopsy and x-rays. There may also be an increased lymphocyte count. Treatment includes surgery for solitary tumors, splenectomy (when the spleen is very large), and chemotherapy. The most common protocol uses prednisone, vincristine, and cyclophosphamide. Doxorubicin is used in some cases. Chemotherapy in relatively healthy ferrets is tolerated very well, but possible side effects include loss of appetite, depression, weakness, vomiting, and loss of whiskers. The white blood cell count must be monitored. Prednisone used alone can work very well for weeks to months, but it may cause resistance to other chemotherapy agents. Alternative treatments include vitamin and Pau d'Arco (a bark extract).

The prognosis for lymphoma in ferrets depends on their health and the location of the cancer. Lymphoma in the mediastinum, spleen, skin, and peripheral lymph nodes has the best prognosis, while lymphoma in the intestine, liver, abdominal lymph nodes, and bone marrow has the worst.

Skin Cancer in Horses

Skin cancer, or neoplasia, is the most common type of cancer diagnosed in horses, accounting for 45 to 80% of all cancers diagnosed. Sarcoids are the most common type of skin neoplasm and are the most common type of cancer overall in horses. Squamous-cell carcinoma is the second-most prevalent skin cancer, followed by melanoma. Squamous-cell carcinoma and melanoma usually occur in horses greater than 9-years-old, while sarcoids commonly affect horses 3 to 6 years old. Surgical biopsy is the method of choice for diagnosis of most equine skin cancers, but is contraindicated for cases of sarcoids. Prognosis and treatment effectiveness varies based on type of cancer, degree of local tissue destruction, evidence of spread to other organs (metastasis) and location of the tumor. Not all cancers metastasize and some can be cured or mitigated by surgical removal of the cancerous tissue or through use of chemotherapeutidrugs.

Sarcoids

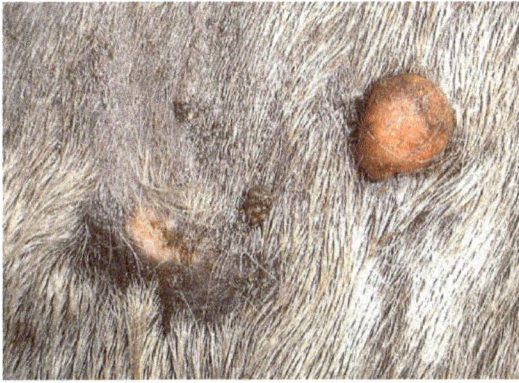

Occult (hairless area at left) and nodular (large round bump at right) forms of equine sarcoids

Sarcoids account for 39.9% of all equine cancers and are the most common cancer diagnosed in horses. There is no breed predilection for developing sarcoids and they can occur at any age, with horses three to six years old being the most common age group and males being slightly more prone to developing the disease. Sarcoids are also more prevalent in certain familial lines, suggesting that there may be a heritable component. Several studies have found an association between the presence of Bovine papillomavirus-1 and 2 and associated viral growth proteins in skin cells with sarcoid formation, but the exact mechanism that controls or induces epidermal proliferation remains unknown. However, high viral loads within cells are strongly correlated with more severe clinical signs and aggressive lesions.

Clinical Signs

The appearance and number of sarcoids can vary, with some horses having single or multiple lesions, usually on the head, legs, ventrum and genitalia or around a wound. The distribution pattern suggests that flies are an important factor in the formation of sarcoids. Sarcoids may resemble warts (verrucous form), small nodules (nodular form), oval hairless or scaly plaques (occult form) or very rarely, large ulcerated masses (fibroblastiform). The occult form usually presents on skin around the mouth, eyes or neck, while nodular and verrucous sarcoids are common on the groin, penile sheath or face. Fibroblastisarcoids have a predilection for the legs, groin, eyelid and sites of previous injury. Multiple forms may also be present on an individual horse (mixed form). Histo-logically, sarcoids are composed of fibroblasts (collagen producing cells) that invade and proliferate within the dermis and sometimes the subcutaneous tissue but do not readily metastasize to other organs. Surgical biopsy can definitively diagnose sarcoids, but there is a significant risk of making sarcoids worse. Therefore, diagnosis based solely on clinical signs, fine-needle aspiration or complete excisional biopsy are safer choices.

Treatment

While sarcoids may spontaneously regress regardless of treatment in some instances, course and duration of disease is highly unpredictable and should be considered on a case-by-case basis taking into account cost of the treatment and severity of clini-cal signs. Surgical removal alone is not effective, with recurrence occurring in 50 to 64% of cases, but removal is often done in conjunction with other treatments. Topi-cal treatment with products containing bloodroot extract (from the plant *Sanguinaria canadensis*) for 7 to 10 days has been reported to be effective in removing small sar-coids, but the salve's caustinature may cause pain and the sarcoid must be in an area where a bandage can be applied. Freezing sarcoids with liquid nitrogen (cryotherapy) is another affordable method, but may result in scarring or depigmentation. Topical ap-plication of the anti-metabolite 5-fluorouracil has also obtained favorable results, but it usually takes 30 to 90 days of repeated application before any effect can be realized. Injection of small sarcoids (usually around the eyes) with the chemotherapeutiagent cisplatin and the immunomodulator BCG have also achieved some success. In one trial, BCG was 69% effective in treating nodular and small fibroblastisarcoids around the eye when repeatedly injected into the lesion and injection with cisplatin was 33% effective overall (mostly in horses with nodular sarcoids). However, BCG treatment carries a risk of allergireaction in some horses and cisplatin has a tendency to leak out of sarcoids during repeated dosing. External beam radiation can also be used on small sarcoids, but is often impractical. There is a chance of sarcoid recurrence for all modalities even after apparently successful treatment. While sarcoids are not fatal, large aggressive tu-mors that destroy surrounding tissue can cause discomfort and loss of function and be resistant to treatment, making euthanasia justifiable in some instances. Sarcoids may be the most common skin-related reason for euthanasia.

Squamous-cell Carcinoma

Squamous-cell carcinoma (SCC) is the most common cancer of the eye, periorbital area and penis, and it is the second most common cancer overall in horses, accounting for 12 to 20% of all cancers diagnosed. While SChas been reported in horses aged 1 to 29-years, most cases occur in 8 to 15-year-old horses, making it the most common neoplasm reported in older horses. Carcinomas are tumors derived from epithelial cells and SCresults from transformation and proliferation of squames, epidermal skin cells that become keratinized. Squamous-cell carcinomas are often solitary, slow-growing tumors that cause extensive local tissue destruction. They can metastasize to other organs, with reported rates as high as 18.6%, primarily to the lymph nodes and lung.

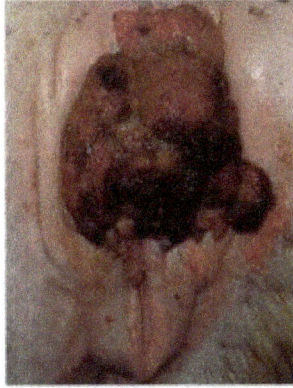

Squamous-cell carcinoma on the vulva of a gray mare, possibly arising from the clitoris. The tumor is ulcerated and has multiple necrotiareas (black spots).

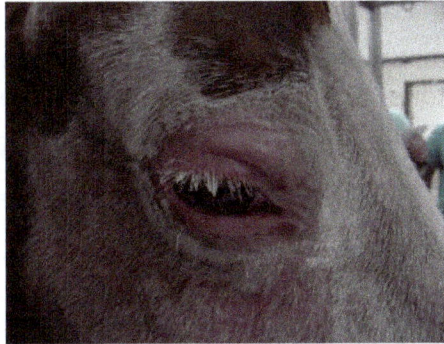

Smooth, raised plaque on upper eyelid of a Paint horse. This horse developed a carcinoma secondary to sunburn (termed solar keratosis carcinoma in situ).

Clinical Signs and Predisposing Factors

Tumors related to squamous-cell carcinoma (SCC) can appear anywhere on the body, but they are most often located in non-pigmented skin near mucocutaneous junctions (where skin meets mucous membranes) such as on the eyelids, around the nostrils, lips, vulva, prepuce, penis or anus. The tumors are raised, fleshy, often ulcerated or infected and may have an irregular surface. Rarely, primary SCdevelops in the esophagus, stomach (non-glandular portion), nasal passages and sinuses, the hard palate, gums, guttural pouches and lung. The eyelid is the most common site, accounting for 40-50% of cases, followed by male (25-10% of cases) and female (10% of cases) genitalia. Horses with lightly pigmented skin, such as those with a gray hair coat or white faces, are especially prone to developing SCC, and some breeds, such as Clydesdales, may have a genetipredisposition. Exposure of light-colored skin to UV light has often been cited as a predisposing factor, but lesions can occur in dark skin and in areas that are not usually exposed to sunlight, such as around the anus. Buildup of smegma ("the bean" in horseman's terms) on the penis is also linked to SCand is thought to be a carcinogen through penile irritation. Pony geldings and work horses are more prone to developing SC on the penis, due to less frequent penile washing when compared to stallions. Equine papillomavirus-2 has also been found within penile SCCs, but has not been determined to cause SCC.

Treatment and Prevention of SCC

Before treatment of squamous-cell carcinoma (SCC) is initiated, evidence of metastasis must be determined either by palpation and aspiration of lymph nodes around the mass or, in smaller horses, radiographs of the thorax. Small tumors found early in the disease process (most frequently on the eyelid) can be treated with cisplatin or radiation with favorable results. For more advanced cases, surgical removal of eye (enucleation), mass or penile amputation can be curative provided all cancerous cells are removed (wide margins obtained) and there is no metastasis. However, young horses (usually geldings less than 8-years-old) that have a hard or "wooden" texture to SCCs on the glans penis have a very poor prognosis for treatment and recovery.

Regular washing of the penis and prepuce in males as well as cleaning the clitoral fossa (the groove around the clitoris) in mares is recommended to remove smegma buildup, which also gives the opportunity for inspection for suspicious growths on the penis or on the vulva.

Melanoma

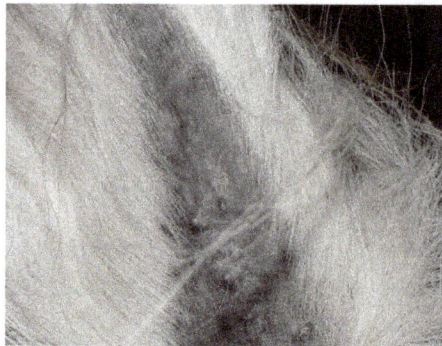

Multiple nodules at the tail-base.

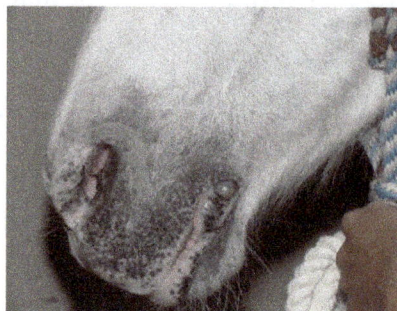

Small nodules at the lip commissure.

Common Sites for Melanoma

Equine Melanoma results from abnormal proliferation and accumulation of mela-nocytes, pigmented cells within the dermis. Gray horses over 6-years-old are espe-cially prone to developing melanoma. The prevalence of melanoma in gray horses over 15 years old has been estimated at 80%. One survey of Camargue-type horses found an overall population prevalence of 31.4%, with prevalence increasing to 67% in horses over 15 years old. Up to 66% of melanomas in gray horses are benign, but melanotitumors in horses with darker hair-coats may be more aggressive and are more often malignant. One retrospective study of cases sent to a referral hospi-tal reported a 14% prevalence of metastatimelanoma within the study population. However, the actual prevalence of metastatimelanoma may be lower due to infre-quent submission of melanotitumors for diagnosis. Common sites for metastasis include lymph nodes, the liver, spleen, lung, skeletal muscle, blood vessels and pa-rotid salivary gland.

Clinical Signs

The most common sites for melanotitumors are on the under-side of the tail near the base, on the prepuce, around the mouth or in the skin over the parotid gland (near the base of the ear). Tumors will initially begin as single, small raised areas that may mul-tiply or coalesce into multi-lobed masses (a process called melanomatosis) over time. Horses under 2-years-old can be born with or acquire benign melanotitumors (called melanocytomas), but these tumors are often located on the legs or trunk, not beneath the tail as in older animals.

Treatment of Melanoma

Treatment of small melanomas is often not necessary, but large tumors can cause dis-comfort and are usually surgically removed. Cisplatin and cryotherapy can be used to treat small tumors less than 3 centimeters, but tumors may reoccur. Cimetidine, a his-tamine stimulator, can cause tumors to regress in some horses, but may take up to 3 months to produce results and multiple treatments may be needed throughout the horse's life. There are few viable treatment options for horses with metastatimelano-ma. However, gene therapy injections utilizing interleukin-12 and 18-encoding DNA plasmids have shown promise in slowing the progression of tumors in patients with metastatimelanoma.

Other Types of Skin Cancer

Lymphoma

Lymphoma is the most common type of blood-related cancer in horses and while it can affect horses of all ages, it typically occurs in horses aged 4–11 years.

Copper Deficiency

Copper deficiency is a very rare hematological and neurological disorder. The neurodegenerative syndrome of copper deficiency has been recognized for some time in ruminant animals, in which it is commonly known as "swayback". Copper is ubiquitous, and daily requirement is low, making acquired copper deficiency very rare. Copper deficiency can manifest in parallel with vitamin B12 and other nutritional deficiencies. The most common cause of copper deficiency is a remote gastrointestinal surgery, such as gastribypass surgery, due to malabsorption of copper, or zintoxicity. On the other hand, Menkes disease is a genetidisorder of copper deficiency involving a wide variety of symptoms that is often fatal. Copper is involved in normalized function of many enzymes, such as cytochrome oxidase, which is complex IV in mitochondrial electron transport chain, ceruloplasmin, Cu/Zn superoxide dismutase, and in amine oxidases. These enzyme catalyze reactions for oxidative phosphorylation, iron transportation, antioxidant and free radical scavenging and neutralization, and neurotransmitter synthesis, respectively. A regular diet contains a variable amount of copper, but may provide 5 mg/day, of which only 20-50% is absorbed. The diet of the elderly may contain a lower copper content than the recommended daily intake. Dietary copper can be found in whole grain cereals, legumes, oysters, organ meats (particularly liver), cherries, dark chocolate, fruits, leafy green vegetables, nuts, poultry, prunes, and soybeans products like tofu. The deficiency in copper can cause many hematological manifestations, such as myelodysplasia, anemia, leukopenia (low white blood cell count) and neutropenia (low count of neutrophils, a type of white blood cell that is often called "the first line of defense" for the immune system). Copper deficiency has long been known for as a cause of myelodysplasia (when a blood profile has indicators of possible future leukemia development), but it was not until recently in 2001 that copper deficiency was associated with neurological manifestations. Some neurological manifestations can be sensory ataxia (irregular coordination due to proprioceptive loss), spasticity, muscle weakness, and more rarely visual loss due to peripheral neuropathy (damage in the peripheral nerves), myelopathy (disease of the spinal cord), and rarely optineuropathy.

Signs and Symptoms

Hematological Presentation

The characteristihematological (blood) effects of copper deficiency are anemia (which may be microcytic, normocytior macrocytic) and neutropenia. Thrombocytopenia (low blood platelets) is unusual.

The peripheral blood and bone marrow aspirate findings in copper deficiency can mimimyelodysplastisyndrome. Bone marrow aspirate in both conditions may show dysplasia of blood cell precursors and the presence of ring sideroblasts (erythoblasts containing multiple iron granules around the nucleus). Unlike most cases of myelo-dysplastisyndrome, the bone marrow aspirate in copper deficiency characteristically shows cytoplasmivacuoles within red and white cell precursors, and karyotyping in cases of copper deficiency does not reveal cytogenetifeatures characteristiof myelodys-plastisyndrome.

Anemia and neutropenia typically resolve within six weeks of copper replacement.

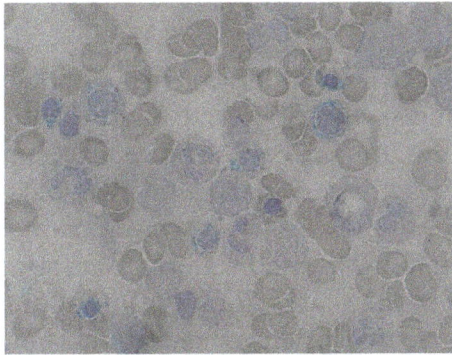

Ring Sideroblast smear 2010-01-13

Neurological Presentation

Copper deficiency can cause a wide variety of neurological problems including, myelopathy, peripheral neuropathy, and optineuropathy.

Myelopathy

Copper deficiency myelopathy in humans was discovered and first described by Schleper and Stuerenburg in 2001. (Schleper B, Stuerenburg HJ. Copper deficiency-associated myelopathy in a 46-year-old woman. J Neurol. 2001 Aug; 248 (8): 705 - 6). They described a patient with a history of gastrectomy and partial coloniresection who presented with severe tetraparesis and painful paraesthesias and who was found on imaging to have dorsomedial cervical cord T2 hyperintensity. Upon further analysis, it was found that the patient had decreased levels of serum coeruloplasmin, serum copper, and CSF copper. The patient was treated with parenteral copper and the patient`s paraesthesias did resolve. Since this discovery, there has been heightened and increasing awareness of copper-deficiency myelopathy and its treatment, and this disorder has been reviewed by Kumar. Sufferers typically present difficulty walking (gait difficulty) caused by sensory ataxia (irregular muscle coordination) due to dorsal column dysfunction or degeneration of the spinal cord (myelopathy). Patients with ataxigait have problems balancing and display an unstable wide walk. They often feel tremors in their torso, causing side way jerks and lunges.

In brain MRI, there is often an increased T2 signalling at the posterior columns of the spinal cord in patients with myelopathy caused by copper deficiency. T2 signalling is often an indicator of some kind of neurodegeneration. There are some changes in the spinal cord MRI involving the thoracicord, the cervical cord or sometimes both. Copper deficiency myelopathy is often compared to subacute combined degeneration (SCD). Subacute combined degeneration is also a degeneration of the spinal cord, but instead vitamin B12 deficiency is the cause of the spinal degeneration. SCD also has the same high T2 signalling intensities in the posterior column as copper deficient patient in MRI imaging.

Peripheral Neuropathy

Another common symptom of copper deficiency is peripheral neuropathy, which is numbness or tingling that can start in the extremities and can sometimes progress radially inward towards the torso. In an Advances in Clinical Neuroscience & Rehabilitation (ACNR) published case report, a 69-year-old patient had progressively worsened neurological symptoms. These symptoms included diminished upper limb reflexes with abnormal lower limb reflexes, sensation to light touch and pin prick was diminished above the waist, vibration sensation was lost in the sternum, and markedly reduced proprioception or sensation about the self's orientation. Many people suffering from the neurological effects of copper deficiency complain about very similar or identical symptoms as the patient. This numbness and tingling poses danger for the elderly because it increases their risk of falling and injuring themselves. Peripheral neuropathy can become very disabling leaving some patients dependent on wheel chairs or walking canes for mobility if there is lack of correct diagnosis. Rarely can copper deficiency cause major disabling symptoms. The deficiency will have to be present for an extensive amount of time until such disabling conditions manifest.

OptiNeuropathy

Some patients suffering from copper deficiency have shown signs of vision and color loss. The vision is usually lost in the peripheral views of the eye. The bilateral vision loss is usually very gradual. An optical coherence tomography (OCT) shows some nerve fiber layer loss in most patients, suggesting the vision loss and color vision loss was secondary to optineuropathy or neurodegeneration.

Causes

Surgery

Bariatrisurgery is a common cause of copper deficiency. Bariatrisurgery, such as gastribypass surgery, is often used for weight control of the morbidly obese. The disruption of the intestines and stomach from the surgery can cause absorption difficulties not only as regards copper, but also for iron and vitamin B12 and many other nutrients. The symptoms of copper deficiency myelopathy may take a long time to develop, sometimes decades before the myelopathy symptoms manifest.

Zinc Toxicity

Increased consumption of zinis another cause of copper deficiency. Zinis often used for the prevention or treatment of common colds and sinusitis (inflammation of sinuses due to an infection), ulcers, sickle cell disease, celiadisease, memory impairment and acne. Zinis found in many common vitamin supplements and is also found in denture creams. Recently, several cases of copper deficiency myeloneuropathy were found to be caused by prolonged use of denture creams containing high quantities of zinc.

Metallizinis the core of all United States currency coins, including copper coated pennies. People who ingest massive amount of coins will have elevated zinlevels, leading to zintoxicity induced copper deficiency and thus displaying neurological symptoms. This was the case for a 57-year-old woman diagnosed with schizophrenia. The woman consumed over 600 coins, and started to show neurological symptoms such as unsteady gait and mild ataxia.

Hereditary Disorders

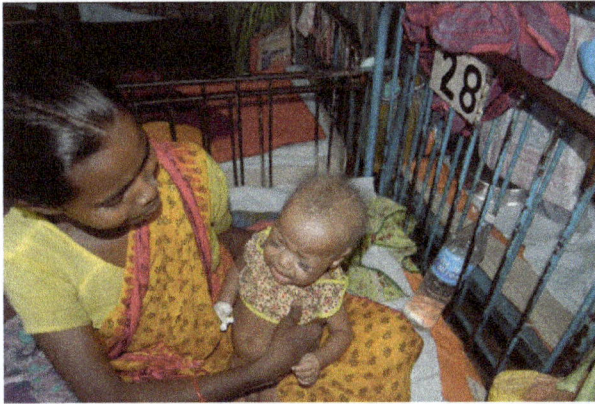

Menkes disease showing symptoms of the sparse, steel colored "kinky hair" and paleness

Menkes disease is a congenital disease that is a cause of copper deficiency. Menkes disease is a hereditary condition caused by a defective gene involved with the metabolism of copper in the body. Menkes disease involves a wide variety of symptoms including floppy muscle tone, seizures, abnormally low temperatures, and a peculiar steel color hair that feels very rough. Menkes disease is usually a fatal disease with most children dying within the first ten years of life.

Other

It is rarely suggested that excess iron supplementation causes copper deficiency myelopathy. Another rarer cause of copper deficiency is Coeliadisease, probably due to malabsorption in the intestines. Still, a large percentage, around 20%, of cases have unknown causes.

Biochemical Etiology

Copper functions as a prosthetigroup, which permits electron transfers in key enzymatipathways like the electron transport chain. Copper is integrated in the enzymes cytochrome oxidase, which is involved in cellular respiration and oxidative phosphorylation, Cu/Zn dismutase, which is involved in antioxidant defense, and many more listed in the table below.

Several Copper Dependent Enzymes and Their Function		
Group	**Enzyme**	**Function**
Oxidases	Flavin-containing amine oxidase	Metabolism of neurotransmitters: noradrenaline, dopamine, serotonin and some dietary amines
	Protein-lysine-6-oxidase (lysyl oxidase)	Connective tissue synthesis- cross-linking of collagen and elastin
	Copper-containing amine oxidase	Metabolism of amines- histamines, putrescine, cadaverine
	Cytochrome oxidase	Oxidative phosphorylation, electron transport in the mitochondrial membrane
	Superoxide dismutase (Cu/Zn dismutase)	Antioxidant and free radical scavenger, oxidizes dangerous superoxides to safer hydrogen peroxide
	Ferroxidase I (ceruloplasmin)	Iron transport-oxidation of Fe^{2+} to Fe^{3+}, copper storage and transport, antioxidant and free radical neutralizer
	Hephaestin (ferroxidase)	Iron transport and oxidation of Fe^{2+} to Fe^{3+} in intestinal cells to enable iron uptake
Monooxygenases	Dopamine beta-monooxygenase	Conversion of dopamine to norepinephrine
	Peptidylglycine monooxygenase	Peptide hormone maturation- amidation of alpha-terminal carboxyliacid group of glycine
	Monophenol monooxygenase (Tyrosinase)	Melanin synthesis
Methylation Cycle	Methionine synthase	Transfer of methyl group from methyltetrahydrofolate to homocysteine to generate methionine for the methylation cycle and tetrahydrofolate for purine synthesis
	Adenosylhomocysteinase (S-Adenosyl-L-homocysteine)	Regeneration of homocysteine from adenosylhomocyeste ine (S-Adenosyl-L-homocysteine) in the methylation cycle

Neurological Etiology

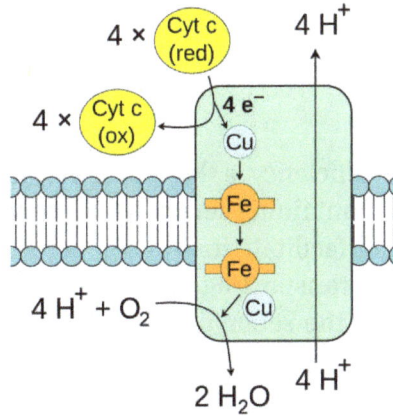

Cytochrome Oxidase mechanism in mitochondrial membrane

Cytochrome Oxidase

There have been several hypotheses about the role of copper and some of its neurological manifestations. Some suggest that disruptions in cytochrome oxidase, also known as Complex IV, of the electron transport chain is responsible for the spinal cord degeneration.

Methylation Cycle

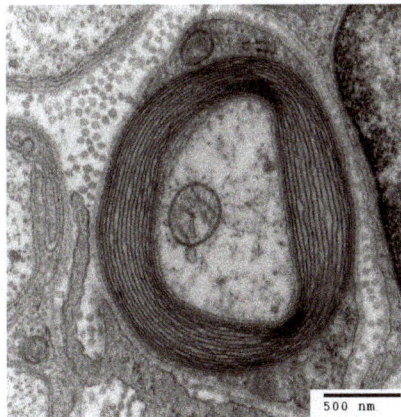

Myelinated neuron

Another hypothesis is that copper deficiency myelopathy is caused by disruptions in the methylation cycle. The methylation cycle causes a transfer of a methyl group (-CH3) from methyltetrahydrofolate to a range of macromolecules by the suspected copper dependent enzyme methionine synthase. This cycle is able to produce purines, which are a component of DNA nucleotide bases, and also myelin proteins. The spinal cord is surrounded by a layer of protective protein coating called myelin. When this methionine synthase enzyme is disrupted, the methylation decreases and myelination of the spinal cord is impaired. This cycle ultimately causes myelopathy.

Hematological Etiology

Iron Transportation

The anemia caused by copper deficiency is thought to be caused by impaired iron transport. Hephaestin is a copper containing ferroxidase enzyme located in the duodenal muscosa that oxidizes iron and facilitate its transfer across the basolateral membrane into circulation. Another iron transporting enzyme is ceruloplasmin. This enzyme is required to mobilize iron from the reticuloendothelial cell to plasma. Ceruloplasmin also oxidizes iron from its ferrous state to the ferriform that is required for iron binding. Impairment in these copper dependent enzymes that transport iron may cause the secondary iron deficiency anemia. Another speculation for the cause of anemia is involving the mitochondrial enzyme cytochrome oxidase (complex IV in the electron transport chain). Studies have shown that animal models with impaired cytochrome oxidase failed to synthesize heme from ferriiron at the normal rate. The lower rate of the enzyme might also cause the excess iron to clump, giving the heme an unusual pattern. This unusual pattern is also known as ringed sideroblastianemia cells.

Cell Growth Halt

The cause of neutropenia is still unclear; however, the arrest of maturing myelocytes, or neutrophil precursors, may cause the neutrophil deficiency.

ZinIntoxication

Zinintoxication may cause anemia by blocking the absorption of copper from the stomach and duodenum. Zinalso upregulates the expression of chelator metallothionein in enterocytes, which are the majority of cells in the intestinal epithelium. Since copper has a higher affinity for metallothionein than zinc, the copper will remain bound inside the enterocyte, which will be later eliminated through the lumen. This mechanism is exploited therapeutically to achieve negative balance in Wilson's disease, which involves an excess of copper.

Treatment

Copper deficiency is a very rare disease and is often misdiagnosed several times by physicians before concluding the deficiency of copper through differential diagnosis (copper serum test and bone marrow biopsy are usually conclusive in diagnosing copper deficiency). On average, patients are diagnosed with copper deficiency around 1.1 years after their first symptoms are reported to a physician. Copper deficiency can be treated with either oral copper supplementation or intravenous copper. If zinintoxication is present, discontinuation of zinmay be sufficient to restore copper levels back to normal, but this usually is a very slow process. People who suffer from zinintoxication will usually have to take copper supplements in addition to ceasing zinconsumption. Hematological manifestations are often quickly restored back to normal. The progression of the neurological symptoms will be stopped by appropriate treatment, but often with residual neurological disability.

Scurvy

Scurvy is a disease resulting from a lack of vitamin C. Early symptoms include weakness, feeling tired, curly hair, and sore arms and legs. Without treatment, decreased red blood cells, gum disease, and bleeding from the skin may occur. As scurvy worsens there can be poor wound healing, personality changes, and finally death from infection or bleeding.

Scurvy is due to not enough vitamin in the diet. It typically takes at least a month of little to no vitamin before symptoms occur. It occurs more commonly in people with mental disorders, unusual eating habits, alcoholism, and old people who live alone. Other risk factors include intestinal malabsorption and dialysis. Humans and certain other animals require vitamin in their diets to make the building blocks for collagen. Diagnosis is typically based on physical signs, X-rays, and improvement after treatment.

Treatment is with vitamin supplements taken by mouth. Improvement often begins in a few days with complete recovery in a few weeks. Sources of vitamin in the diet include citrus fruit and a number of vegetables such as tomatoes and potatoes. Cooking often decreases vitamin in foods.

Scurvy is currently rare. It occurs more often in the developing world in association with malnutrition. Rates among refugees are reported at 5% to 45%. Scurvy was described as early as the time of ancient Egypt. It was a limiting factor in long distance sea travel, often killing large numbers of people. A Scottish surgeon in the Royal Navy, James Lind, was the first to prove it could be treated with citrus fruit in a 1753 publication. His experiments represented the first controlled trial. It took another 40 years before the British Navy began giving out lemon juice routinely.

Signs and Symptoms

Early symptoms are malaise and lethargy. Even earlier might be a pain in a section of the gums which interferes with digestion. After 1–3 months, patients develop shortness of breath and bone pain. Myalgias may occur because of reduced carnitine production. Other symptoms include skin changes with roughness, easy bruising and petechiae, gum disease, loosening of teeth, poor wound healing, and emotional changes (which may appear before any physical changes). Dry mouth and dry eyes similar to Sjögren's syndrome may occur. In the late stages, jaundice, generalized edema, oliguria, neuropathy, fever, convulsions, and eventual death are frequently seen.

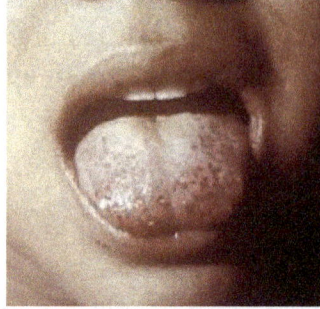

A child presenting a "scorbutitongue" due to what proved to be a vitamin deficiency.

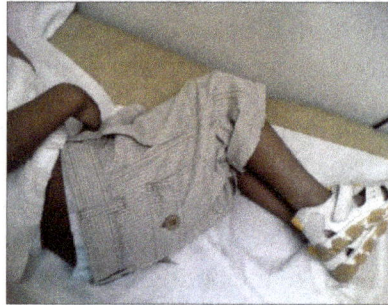

A child with scurvy in flexion posture.

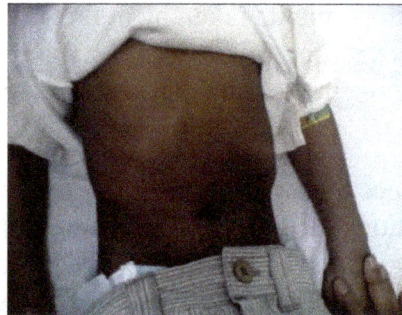

Photo of the chest cage with pectus excavatum and scorbutirosaries.

Cause

Scurvy or subclinical scurvy is caused by the lack of vitamin C. In modern Western societies, scurvy is rarely present in adults, although infants and elderly people are affected. Virtually all commercially available baby formulas contain added vitamin C. Human breast milk contains sufficient vitamin C, if the mother has an adequate intake.

Scurvy is one of the accompanying diseases of malnutrition (other such micronutrient deficiencies are beriberi or pellagra) and thus is still widespread in areas of the world depending on external food aid. Though rare, there are also documented cases of scurvy due to poor dietary choices by people living in industrialized nations.

Pathogenesis

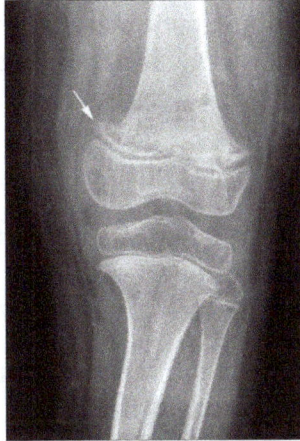

X-ray of the lower and upper limbs (arrow indicates scurvy line).

Ascorbiacid is needed for a variety of biosynthetipathways, by accelerating hydroxylation and amidation reactions. In the synthesis of collagen, ascorbiacid is required as a cofactor for prolyl hydroxylase and lysyl hydroxylase. These two enzymes are responsible for the hydroxylation of the proline and lysine amino acids in collagen. Hydroxyproline and hydroxylysine are important for stabilizing collagen by cross-linking the propeptides in collagen. Defective collagen fibrillogenesis impairs wound healing. Collagen is an important part of bone, so bone formation is affected. Defective connective tissue leads to fragile capillaries, resulting in abnormal bleeding. Untreated scurvy is invariably fatal.

Prevention

Scurvy can be prevented by a diet that includes vitamin C-rich foods such as sweet peppers, guava, blackcurrants, parsley, broccoli, and kiwifruit. Other sources rich in vitamin are fruits such as papaya, strawberries and oranges or lemons. It is also found in vegetables, such as brussels sprouts, cabbage, spinach, and potatoes. Some fruits and vegetables not high in vitamin may be pickled in lemon juice, which is high in vitamin C. Though redundant in the presence of a balanced diet, various nutritional supplements are available that provide ascorbiacid well in excess of that required to prevent scurvy.

Some animal products, including liver, Muktuk (whale skin), oysters, and parts of the central nervous system, including the brain, spinal cord, and adrenal medulla, contain large amounts of vitamin C, and can even be used to treat scurvy. Fresh meat from animals which make their own vitamin (which most animals do) contains enough vitamin to prevent scurvy, and even partly treat it. In some cases (notably in French soldiers eating fresh horse meat), it was discovered that meat alone, even partly cooked meat, could alleviate scurvy. In other cases, a meat-only diet could cause scurvy.

Scott's 1902 expedition used lightly fried seal meat and liver, whereby complete recovery from incipient scurvy was reported to take less than two weeks.

History

Scurvy was documented as a disease by Hippocrates, and Egyptians have recorded its symptoms as early as 1550 BCE. The knowledge that consuming foods containing vitamin is a cure for scurvy has been repeatedly rediscovered and forgotten into the early 20th century.

Early Modern Era

In the 13th century, the Crusaders frequently suffered from scurvy. In the 1497 expedition of Vasco de Gama, the curative effects of citrus fruit were already known and confirmed by Pedro Álvares Cabral and his crew in 1507.

The Portuguese also planted fruit trees and vegetables in Saint Helena, a stopping point for homebound voyages from Asia, and left their sick, suffering from scurvy and other ailments to be taken home, if they recovered, by the next ship.

Unfortunately, these travel accounts have not stopped further maritime tragedies caused by scurvy, first because of the lack of communication between travelers and those responsible for their health and also because fruits and vegetables could not be kept for long on ships.

In 1536, the French explorer Jacques Cartier, exploring the St. Lawrence River, used the local natives' knowledge to save his men who were dying of scurvy. He boiled the needles of the arbor vitae tree (Eastern White Cedar) to make a tea that was later shown to contain 50 mg of vitamin per 100 grams. Such treatments were not available aboard ship, where the disease was most common.

Between 1500 and 1800, it has been estimated that scurvy killed at least two million sailors. Jonathan Lamb wrote: "In 1499, Vasco da Gama lost 116 of his crew of 170; In 1520, Magellan lost 208 out of 230;...all mainly to scurvy."

In 1593, Admiral Sir Richard Hawkins advocated drinking orange and lemon juice as a means of preventing scurvy.

In 1614 John Woodall, Surgeon General of the East India Company, published "The Surgion's Mate" as a handbook for apprentice surgeons aboard the company's ships. He repeated the experience of mariners that the cure for scurvy was fresh food or, if not available, oranges, lemons, limes and tamarinds. He was, however, unable to explain the reason why and his assertion had no impact on the opinion of the influential physicians who ran the medical establishment that it was a digestive complaint.

18th Century

A 1707 handwritten book by Mrs. Ebot Mitchell discovered in a house in Hasfield, Gloucestershire, contains a "Recp.t for the Scurvy" that consisted of extracts from various plants mixed with a plentiful supply of orange juice, white wine or beer.

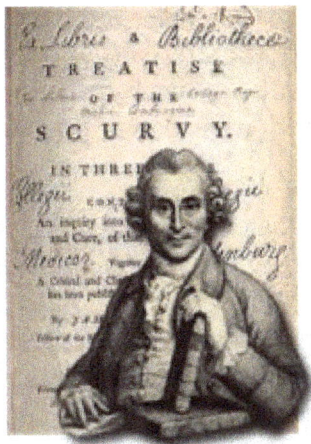

James Lind, a pioneer in the field of scurvy prevention

In 1734, the Leiden-based physician Johann Bachstrom published a book on scurvy in which he stated that "scurvy is solely owing to a total abstinence from fresh vegetable food, and greens; which is alone the primary cause of the disease" and urged the use of fresh fruit and vegetables as a cure.

However, it was not until 1747 that James Lind formally demonstrated that scurvy could be treated by supplementing the diet with citrus fruit, in the first ever clinical trial. In 1753, Lind published *A Treatise of the Scurvy,* in which he explained the details of his clinical trial, but it occupied only a few paragraphs in a work that was long and complex and had little impact. In fact, Lind himself never actively promoted lemon juice as a single 'cure'. He shared medical opinion at the time that scurvy had multiple causes – notable hard work, bad water and the consumption of salt meat in a damp atmosphere which inhibited healthful perspiration and normal excretion - and therefore required multiple solutions. He was also side-tracked by the possibilities of producing a concentrated 'rob' of lemon juice by boiling it. Unfortunately this process destroyed the vitamin and was unsuccessful.

During the 18th century, disease killed more British sailors than enemy action. It was mainly by scurvy that George Anson, in his celebrated voyage of 1740–1744, lost nearly two-thirds of his crew (1300 out of 2000) within the first ten months of the voyage. The Royal Navy enlisted 184,899 sailors during the Seven Years' War; 133,708 of these were "missing" or died by disease, and scurvy was the leading cause.

Although throughout this period sailors and naval surgeons were increasingly convinced that citrus fruits could cure scurvy, the classically trained physicians who ran the medical establishment dismissed this evidence as mere anecdote which did not conform to current theories of disease. Literature championing the cause of citrus juice therefore had no practical impact. Medical theory was based on the assumption that scurvy was a disease of internal putrefaction brought on by faulty digestion caused by the hardships of life at sea and the naval diet. Although this basiidea was given different emphases by successive theorists, the remedies they advocated (and which the navy accepted) amounted to little more than the consumption of 'fizzy drinks' to activate the digestive system, the most extreme of which was the regular consumption of 'elixir of vitriol' – sulphuriacid taken with spirits and barley water and laced with spices.

In 1764, a new variant appeared. Advocated by Dr David McBride and Sir John Pringle, Surgeon General of the Army and later President of the Royal Society, this idea was that scurvy was the result of a lack of 'fixed air' in the tissues which could be prevented by drinking infusions of malt and wort whose fermentation within the body would stimulate digestion and restore the missing gases. These ideas receiving wide and influential backing, when James Cook set off to circumnavigate the world (1768–1771) in HM Bark *Endeavour*, malt and wort were top of the list of the remedies he was ordered to investigate. The others were beer, sour crout and Lind's 'rob'. The list did not include lemons.

Cook did not lose a single man to scurvy, and his report came down in favour of malt and wort, although it is now clear that the reason for the health of his crews on this and other voyages was Cook's regime of shipboard cleanliness, enforced by strict discipline, as well as frequent replenishment of fresh food and green stuffs. Another rule implemented by Cook was his prohibition of the consumption of salt fat skimmed from the ship's copper boiling pans, then a common practice in the Navy. In contact with air the copper formed compounds that prevented the absorption of vitamins by the intestines.

The first major long distance expedition that experienced virtually no scurvy was that of the Spanish naval officer Alessandro Malaspina, 1789–1794. Malaspina's medical officer, Pedro González, was convinced that fresh oranges and lemons were essential for preventing scurvy. Only one outbreak occurred, during a 56-day trip across the open sea. Five sailors came down with symptoms, one seriously. After three days at Guam all five were healthy again. Spain's large empire and many ports of call made it easier to acquire fresh fruit.

Although towards the end of the century MacBride's theories were being challenged, the medical establishment in Britain remained wedded to the notion that scurvy was a disease of internal 'putrefaction' and the Sick and Hurt Board, run by administrators, felt obliged to follow its advice. Within the Royal Navy however opinion - strengthened by first-hand experience of the use of lemon juice at the siege of Gibraltar and during Admiral Rodney's expedition to the Caribbean - had become increasingly convinced of its efficacy. This was reinforced by the writings of experts like Gilbert Blane and Thomas Trotter and by the reports of up-and-coming naval commanders.

With the coming of war in 1793, the need to eliminate scurvy acquired a new urgency. But the first initiative came not from the medical establishment but from the admirals. Ordered to lead an expedition against Mauritius, Rear Admiral Gardner was uninterested in the wort, malt and elixir of vitriol which were still being issued to ships of the Royal Navy, and demanded that he be supplied with lemons to counteract scurvy on the voyage. Members of the Sick and Hurt Board, recently augmented by two practical naval surgeons, supported the request and the Admiralty ordered that it be done. There was however a last minute change of plan. The expedition against Mauritius was cancelled. On 2 May 1794, only HMS *Suffolk* and two sloops under Commodore Peter Rainier sailed for the east with an outward bound convoy, but the warships were fully supplied with lemon juice and the sugar with which it had to be mixed. Then in March 1795, came astonishing news. *Suffolk* had arrived in India after a four-month voyage without a trace of scurvy and with a crew that was healthier than when it set out.

The effect was immediate. Fleet commanders clamoured also to be supplied with lemon juice and by June the Admiralty acknowledged the groundswell of demand in the navy had agreed to a proposal from the Sick and Hurt Board that lemon juice and sugar should in future be issued as a daily ration to the crews of all warships.

It took a few years before the method of distribution to all ships in the fleet had been perfected and the supply of the huge quantities of lemon juice required to be secured, but by 1800, the system was in place and functioning. This led to a remarkable health improvement among the sailors and consequently played a critical role in gaining the advantage in naval battles against enemies who had yet to introduce the measures.

19th Century

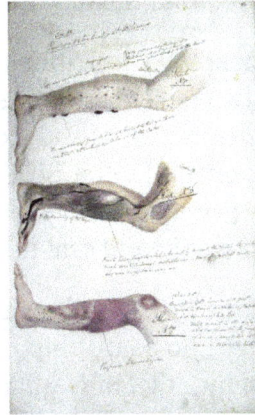

Page from the journal of Henry Walsh Mahon showing the effects of scurvy, from his time aboard HM Convict Ship Barrosa. 1841/2

The surgeon-in-chief of Napoleon's army at the Siege of Alexandria (1801), Baron Dominique-Jean Larrey, wrote in his memoirs that the consumption of horse meat helped the French to curb an epidemiof scurvy. The meat was cooked but was freshly obtained from young horses bought from Arabs and was nevertheless effective. This helped to start the 19th-century tradition of horse meat consumption in France.

Lauchlin Rose patented a method used to preserve citrus juice without alcohol in 1867, creating a concentrated drink known as Rose's lime juice. The Merchant Shipping Act established in the year 1867 required all ships of the Royal Navy and Merchant Navy to provide a daily lime ration to sailors to prevent scurvy. The product became nearly ubiquitous, hence the term "limey", first for British sailors, then for English immigrants within the former British colonies (particularly America, New Zealand and South Africa), and finally, in old American slang, all British people.

The plant *Cochlearia officinalis*, also known as "Common Scurvygrass", acquired its common name from the observation that it cured scurvy, and it was taken on board ships in dried bundles or distilled extracts. Its very bitter taste was usually disguised with herbs and spices; however, this did not prevent scurvygrass drinks and sandwiches becoming a popular fad in the UK until the middle of the nineteenth century, when citrus fruits became more readily available.

West Indian limes began to supplement lemons when Spain's alliance with France against Britain in the NapoleoniWars made the supply of Mediterranean lemons problematiand because they were more easily obtained from Britain's Caribbean colonies and were believed to be more effective because they were more acidic, and it was the acid, not the (then-unknown) Vitamin that was believed to cure scurvy. In fact, the West Indian limes were significantly lower in Vitamin than the previous lemons and further were not served fresh but rather as lime juice, which had been exposed to light and air and piped through copper tubing, all of which significantly reduced the Vitamin C. Indeed, a 1918 animal experiment using representative samples of the Navy and Merchant Marine's lime juice showed that it had virtually no antiscorbutipower at all.

The belief that scurvy was fundamentally a nutritional deficiency, best treated by consumption of fresh food, particularly fresh citrus or fresh meat, was not universal in the 19th and early 20th centuries, and thus sailors and explorers continued to suffer from scurvy into the 20th century. For example, the Belgian AntarctiExpedition of 1897–1899 became seriously affected by scurvy when its leader Adrien de Gerlache initially discouraged his men from eating penguin and seal meat.

In the Royal Navy's Arctiexpeditions in the 19th century it was widely believed that scurvy was prevented by good hygiene on board ship, regular exercise, and maintaining the morale of the crew, rather than by a diet of fresh food. Navy expeditions continued to be plagued by scurvy even while fresh (not jerked or tinned) meat was well known as a practical antiscorbutiamong civilian whalers and explorers in the Arctic. Even cooking fresh meat did not entirely destroy its antiscorbutiproperties, especially as many cooking methods failed to bring all the meat to high temperature.

The confusion is attributed to a number of factors:

- while *fresh* citrus (particularly lemons) cured scurvy, lime *juice* that had been exposed to light, air and copper tubing did not – thus undermining the theory that citrus cured scurvy;

- fresh meat (especially organ meat and raw meat, consumed in arctiexploration) also cured scurvy, undermining the theory that fresh vegetable matter was essential to preventing and curing scurvy;

- increased marine speed via steam shipping, and improved nutrition on land, reduced the incidence of scurvy – and thus the ineffectiveness of copper-piped lime juice compared to fresh lemons was not immediately revealed.

In the resulting confusion, a new hypothesis was proposed, following the new germ theory of disease – that scurvy was caused by ptomaine, a waste product of bacteria, particularly in tainted tinned meat.

Infantile scurvy emerged in the late 19th century because children were being fed pasteurized cow's milk, particularly in the urban upper class – the pasteurization killed bacteria but also destroyed vitamin C. This was eventually resolved by supplementing with onion juice or cooked potatoes.

20th Century

At the time Robert Falcon Scott made his first expedition (1901–1904) to the Antarctiin the early 20th century, the prevailing theory was that scurvy was caused by "ptomaine poisoning", particularly in tinned meat. However, Scott discovered that a diet of fresh meat from Antarctiseals cured scurvy before any fatalities occurred.

In 1907, an animal model which would eventually help to isolate and identify the "antiscorbutifactor" was discovered. Axel Holst and Theodor Frølich, two Norwegian physicians studying shipboard beriberi contracted aboard ship's crews in the Norwegian Fishing Fleet, wanted a small test mammal to substitute for the pigeons then used in beriberi research. They fed guinea pigs their test diet of grains and flour, which had earlier produced beriberi in their pigeons, and were surprised when classiscurvy resulted instead. This was a serendipitous choice of animal. Until that time, scurvy had not been observed in any organism apart from humans and had been considered an exclusively human disease. (Some birds are susceptible to scurvy, but pigeons are unaffected by scurvy, as they produce vitamin C.) Holst and Frølich found they could cure scurvy in guinea pigs with the addition of various fresh foods and extracts. This discovery of an animal experimental model for scurvy, which was made even before the essential idea of "vitamins" in foods had been put forward, has been called the single most important piece of vitamin research.

Vilhjalmur Stefansson, an arctiexplorer who had lived among the Inuit, proved that the all-meat diet they consumed did not lead to vitamin deficiencies. He participated in a study in New York's Bellevue Hospital in February 1928, where he and a companion ate only meat for a year while under close medical observation, yet remained in good health.

In 1927, Hungarian biochemist Szent-Györgyi isolated a compound he called "hexuroniacid". Szent-Györgyi suspected hexuroniacid, which he had isolated from adrenal glands, to be the antiscorbutiagent, but he could not prove it without an animal-deficiency model. In 1932, the connection between hexuroniacid and scurvy was finally proven by American researcher Charles Glen King of the University of Pittsburgh. King's laboratory was given some hexuroniacid by Szent-Györgyi and soon established that it was the sought-after anti-scorbutiagent. Because of this, hexuroniacid was subsequently renamed *ascorbiacid.*

21st Century

In the 2010s scurvy hasn't entirely disappeared from developed countries and rates while still very low, are increasing in the United Kingdom according to NHS Digital. Several cases were also reported in Westmead Hospital, Sydney, Australia.

Human Trials

Notable human dietary studies of experimentally induced scurvy have been conducted on conscientious objectors during WWII in Britain and on Iowa state prisoner "volunteers" in the late 1960s. These studies both found that all obvious symptoms of scurvy previously induced by an experimental scorbutidiet with extremely low vitamin content could be completely reversed by additional vitamin supplementation of only 10 mg per day. In these experiments, no clinical difference was noted between men given 70 mg vitamin per day (which produced blood levels of vitamin of about 0.55 mg/dl, about 1/3 of tissue saturation levels), and those given 10 mg per day (which produced lower blood levels). Men in the prison study developed the first signs of scurvy about 4 weeks after starting the vitamin C-free diet, whereas in the British study, six to eight months were required, possibly because the subjects were pre-loaded with a 70 mg/day supplement for six weeks before the scorbutidiet was fed.

Men in both studies on a diet devoid or nearly devoid of vitamin had blood levels of vitamin too low to be accurately measured when they developed signs of scurvy, and in the Iowa study, at this time were estimated (by labeled vitamin dilution) to have a body pool of less than 300 mg, with daily turnover of only 2.5 mg/day.

Other Animals

Scurvy does not occur in most animals as they can make their own vitamin C. However, humans and other higher primates (the simians—monkeys and apes—and tarsiers), guinea pigs, most or all bats, and some species of birds and fish lack an enzyme (L-gulonolactone oxidase) necessary for such synthesis and must obtain vitamin through their diet. The gene for L-gulonolactone oxidase is still present in the human genome, but deactivated by DNA mutations.

Almost all plant and animal species synthesize vitamin C. Notable mammalian exceptions include most or all of the order Chiroptera (bats), and one of the two major primate suborders, the "Anthropoidea" (Haplorrhini) which include tarsiers, monkeys, and apes, including human beings. The Strepsirrhini (non-tarsier prosimians) can make their own vitamin C, and these include lemurs, lorises, pottos, and galagos. Ascorbiacid is also not synthesized by at least two species of Caviidae, the capybara and the guinea pig. There are known species of birds and fish that do not synthesize their own Vitamin C. All species that do not synthesize ascorbate require it in the diet. Deficiency causes scurvy in humans, and somewhat similar symptoms in other animals.

Name

In babies, scurvy is sometimes referred to as Barlow's disease, named after Thomas Barlow, a British physician who described it in 1883. However, Barlow's disease may also refer to mitral valve prolapse.

Berserk Llama Syndrome

Berserk llama syndrome or berserk male syndrome (as it is more pronounced in males) is a psychological condition suffered by human-raised llamas and alpacas that can cause them to exhibit dangerously aggressive behavior toward humans. The term has been overused, however, and is sometimes inappropriately applied to llamas with aggressive personalities that are not truly "berserk".

The condition is a result of the llama imprinting on its human handlers to such a degree that it considers them to be fellow llamas. Imprinting can be caused by bottle feeding and by isolation from other llamas. Adult male inter-llama interaction can be rough, including chest-ramming and biting, and they are strongly territorial. Male llamas suffering from this condition become dangerous when this behavior is directed toward humans and they usually have to be euthanised. Female llamas can also suffer from berserk llama syndrome but their behavior is usually limited to spitting and difficult handling.

Berserk llama syndrome can be prevented in males through castration before puberty.

Panzootic

A panzooti is an epizooti(an outbreak of an infectious disease of animals) that spreads across a large region (for example a continent), or even worldwide. The equivalent in human populations is called a pandemic.

A panzootican start when three conditions have been met:

- the emergence of a disease new to the population.

- the agent infects a species and causes serious illness.

- the agent spreads easily and sustainably among animals.

A disease or condition is not a panzootimerely because it is widespread or kills a large number of animals; it must also be infectious. For example, cancer is responsible for a large number of deaths but is not considered a panzootibecause the disease is, generally speaking, not infectious. Unlike an epizootic, a panzooticovers all or nearly all species over a large surface area (ex. rabies, anthrax). Typically an enzootior an epizootic, or their cause, may act as a potential preparatory factor .

Causes of Spread and Environmental Influences

Contagion and infection by far play the biggest role in the dissemination and spread of epizootiand panzootidiseases. These include virulent (ex. Cattle Plague), septi(can be caused in the change in food quality), parasiti(ex. Scabies), and miasmatiinfections (ex. Typhoid Fever). Many claim that an accidental morbificause, which infects a great amount of animals which ceases activity after a prolonged time period.

Certain factors come into play in the spread of certain panzootidiseases, as can be seen with Batrachochytrium dendrobatidis. This infection seems to be sensitive to external conditions, particularly the environments temperature and moisture. These factors leads to limitations on where the diseases can thrive, acting almost as its 'climate niche'.

Examples

Persistence of H5N1 Avian Influenza

H5N1, the highly pathogenistrain of influenza, was first detected in the goose population of Gaungdong, China in 1996.

In February 2004, avian influenza virus was detected in birds in Vietnam, increasing fears of the emergence of new variant strains. It is feared that if the avian influenza virus combines with a human influenza virus (in a bird or a human), the new subtype created could be both highly contagious and highly lethal.

In October 2005, cases of the avian flu (the deadly strain H5N1) were identified in Turkey. EU Health Commissioner Markos Kyprianou said: "We have received now confirmation that the virus found in Turkey is an avian flu H5N1 virus. There is a direct relationship with viruses found in Russia, Mongolia and China." Cases of bird flu were also identified shortly thereafter in Romania, and then Greece. Possible cases of the virus have also been found in Croatia, Bulgaria and in the United Kingdom. However, by the end of October only 67 people had died as a result of H5N1 which was atypical of previous influenza pandemics.

The enzooicity of H5N1 in birds, poultry in particular, has led to a major panzootic. As of 2012, there was an estimated 400 million birds killed from infection of the H5N1 strain of influenza. Studies have shown that H5N1 is very well adapted to domestiduck and geese, making them key in controlling the H5N1 strain and preventing future panzootievents.

Presently, the highly pathogeniAsian strain of Avian Influenza is still continuing to kill poultry and wild birds alike on panzootiscales. The persistence of such a pathogen in the environment would only lead to a further continuation of panzootiscale eliminations of birds. To try to control this, scientists did research involving the shed feathers of domestiducks to test the prevalence of H5N1. Although viral persistence was notably found within drinking water and feces, the feathers exhibited the most remaining H5N1 strain for up to 160 days. The persistence exhibited through the feathers indicates the potential for environmental contamination of not only H5N1, but also other untested viruses.

White Nose Syndrome in Bats

White Nose Syndrome (WNS) is a rapidly spreading fungal infection responsible for killing millions of bats within the past 9 years.*Geomyces-destructans* is the causative fungal agent of the characteristiskin lesions seen on the exposed skin, particularly on wings and nose, and in the hair follicles of affected bats. WNS has only recently been discovered, in Howe's Cave, New York during the winter of 2006-2007, but affects 25% of the hibernating species. Six species of bats have been fatally effected by this panzootic; big brown bat, small-footed bat, little brown bat, northern long-eared bat, Indiana bat, and tricolored bat, and current bat population surveys suggest a 2-year population decline in excess of 75%. The geographical range of WNS has spread throughout 33 states, and 4 Canadian provinces.

The mechanism of how the infection on the skin kills bats is unclear. However, the outward cause of mortality of the infected bats depends on the stage and severity of the bat. Infected bats commonly die from starvation over winter, and can suffer from lasting damage to the wing membranes and impair summer foraging if survived the winter. One of the most abundant bat species in eastern North America, the little brown bat (*Myotis lucifugus*), could disappear from this region within 16 years.

Severely infected bats emerge prematurely from hibernation, and if they survive long enough and enter a different hibernaculum, the likelihood of transmission isprobably high, because they presumably carry a large load of fungal spores. Transmission of the infection is either physically from bat-to-bat contact, or from and hibernaculum-to-bat, through the exposure to spores of *Geomyces- destructans* that were present on a roosting substrate.

Newcastle Disease in Pigeons

Newcastle disease is a contagious bird disease affecting many domestiand wild avian species. The disease is contagious through immediate contact between healthy birds and the bodily discharges of infected birds. This includes transmission through droppings, secretions from the nose, mouth and eyes. Newcastle disease spreads quickly among birds kept in captivity, such as commercially raised chickens. Symptoms include sneezing, gasping for air, nasal discharge, coughing, greenish and watery diarrhea, nervousness, depression, muscular tremors, drooping wings, twisting of head and neck, circling, complete paralysis, partial to complete drop in egg production and thin-shelled eggs, swelling of the tissues around the eyes and in the neck, and sudden death.

Newcastle disease was first identified in Java, Indonesia, in 1926, and in 1927, in Newcastle upon Tyne, England (whence it got its name). However, it may have been prevalent as early as 1898, when a disease wiped out all the domestifowl in northwest Scotland. Its effects are most notable in domestipoultry due to their high susceptibility and the potential for severe impacts of an epizootion the poultry industries. It is endemito many countries. The emergence and spread of new genotypes across the world represents a significant threat to poultry. This suggests that the disease is continuously evolving, leading to more diversity (Miller et al., 2009).

Unfortunately, little has been done to comprehend the procedure and advancement of new genotypes (Alexander et al., 2012). Recent vNDV have been characterized as isolates and offer evidence which proposes an emergence of a fifth panzootiinitiated by highly related vNDV isolates from Indonesia, Israel and Pakistan. These virus strains are related to older strains from wild birds. This suggests that unknown reservoirs harbor new vNDV isolates capable of additional panzootics.

No treatment for NDV exists, but the use of prophylactivaccines and sanitary measures reduces the likelihood of outbreaks.

Chytrid Fungus in Amphibian Populations

Chytridiomycosis caused by a chytrid fungus is a deadly fungal disease that has wiped out 30 amphibian species across the globe and has sent overall amphibian populations in decline. The fungus *Batrachochytrium dendrobatidis* can be found on every continent with fertile soil and has contributed to the loss of some species of frogs and salamanders. In fact, it is estimated that 287 species of amphibians are infected with this disease in over 35 countries. These countries tend to have varied or tropical climates like those found in Central America, South America, and Africa with optimal climate conditions ranging from 17 degree Celsius to 23 degrees Celsius for the fungus to thrive.

The first reported instance of the chytrid fungus was in 1998 which was found on the skin of amphibians. Since amphibians absorb essential nutrients through their skin, the fungus attaches itself to the amphibian, suffocates the amphibian, and enters the blood stream of the organism. Some symptoms that are prevalent in affected species include lethargy and loss of equilibrium and begin to die 21 days after infection. Frogs that have died and are examined show high density of the fungal spores in keratinized areas of the body such as the pelvis, mouth, and underbelly.

The fungus is spread through the transportation of amphibious species by humans. Infected amphibians that have escaped or are released into the wild can carry the fungus and therefore invade the surrounding habitats of local species that are not immune to the disease. Species like the American Bullfrog and African Clawed Frog can carry this disease without experiencing symptoms or death; these kinds of species are usually to blame for the spread of the disease in undeveloped habitats.

Some characteristics of amphibians that are more likely to be susceptible to the disease are the lack of various developed microbiota that live and breed on the dermis of the species as well the underdeveloped immune system in specifiamphibians. Species that tend to breed in flowing water which washes away the microbiota from the skin of amphibians are more likely to become infected. Organizations across the world have tried to implement rules and regulations for the transportation of amphibians across borders to prevent the continued decline of amphibians however progress has been slow. To add to the slow progress, the only cure that exists for chytrid fungus is found within laboratories for amphibians in captivity. Because of this, there is no known way for eradicating the disease in the wild.

Transport Tetany

Transport tetany is a disease which occurs in cows and ewes after the stress of prolonged transport in crowded, hot and poorly ventillated vehicles. It is commonly seen in animals in late pregnancy and those transported to slaughter in crowded, hot, and poorly ventillated vehicles. The disease is generally fatal, even with treatment, unless detected early. It is also known as "transit tetany", "railroad disease", "railroad sickness", or "staggers".

Early clinical signs include restlessness, excitement, trismus, grinding of teeth, staggering gait and later paddling of hind legs. Rumen hypomotility, gastrointestinal stasis and anorexia develop. Also may develop tachycardia and rapid, labored respiration. If not recovered, cattle die, often after a coma.

It may also happen in horses.

Epilepsy in Animals

Seizures are caused by abnormal bursts of electrical activity in the brain. They can start and stop very abruptly and last any amount of time from a few seconds to a few minutes. Epilepsy can occur in animals other than humans. Canine epilepsy is often genetibut epilepsy in cats and other pets is rarer, likely because there is no hereditary component to epilepsy in these animals.

Characteristics

Epilepsy is most commonly recognised by involuntary movements of the head and limbs, however other characteristics include salivation, lack of bodily functions and anxiety. Animals often lose consciousness and are not aware of their surroundings.

Handling Seizures

Watching an animal or person have a seizure can be quite frightening. There is not much that can be done during a seizure except to ensure that you remain calm and do not leave the animal alone. If your pet is having a seizure it is important to make sure they are laying down on the floor away from any water, stairs or other animals. When an animal has a seizure, do not try to grab their tongue or clear their mouth as there is a high chance you will be bitten; contrary to popular myth, neither humans nor animals can "swallow their tongue" during a seizure so it is safest to stay well away from their mouth during one. Timing seizures is also crucial; if a seizure lasts for more than 5 minutes or your pet is having multiple seizures per day then a veterinary doctor should be contacted. Take notes of seizures - what time they occur, how often and any other specifiinformation which can be passed onto the vet or emergency animal clinic.

Canine Epilepsy

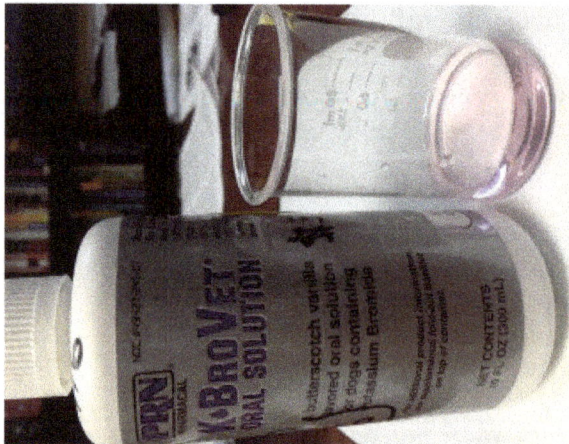

A bottle of PRN Pharmaceutical Company (Pensacola, FL) *K·BroVet* veterinary pharmaceutical potassium bromide oral solution (250 mg / mL). The product is intended to be used in dogs, primarily as an antiepilepti(to stop seizures).

In dogs, epilepsy is often an inherited condition. The incidence of epilepsy/seizures in the general dog population is estimated to be between 0.5% and 5.7%. In certain breeds, {{such as the Belgian Shepherd varieties}}, the incidence may be much higher.

Diagnosis

There are three types of epilepsy in dogs: reactive, secondary, and primary. Reactive epileptiseizures are caused by metaboliissues, such as low blood sugar or kidney or liver failure. Epilepsy attributed to brain tumor, stroke or other trauma is known as secondary or symptomatiepilepsy.

There is no known cause for primary or idiopathiepilepsy, which is only diagnosed by eliminating other possible causes for the seizures. Dogs with idiopathiepilepsy experience their first seizure between the ages of one and three. However, the age at diagnosis is only one factor in diagnosing canine epilepsy, as one study found cause for seizures in one-third of dogs between the ages of one and three, indicating secondary or reactive rather than primary epilepsy.

A veterinarian's initial work-up for a dog presenting with a history of seizures may include a physical and neurological exam, a complete blood count, serum chemistry profile, urinalysis, bile tests, and thyroid function tests. These tests verify seizures and may determine cause for reactive or secondary epilepsy. Veterinarians may also request that dog owners keep a "seizure log" documenting the timing, length, severity, and recovery of each seizure, as well as dietary or environmental changes.

Treatment

Many antiepileptidrugs are used for the management of canine epilepsy. Oral phenobarbital, in particular, and imepitoin are considered to be the most effective antiepileptidrugs and usually used as 'first line' treatment. Other anti-epileptics such as zonisamide, primidone, gabapentin, pregabalin, sodium valproate, felbamate and topiramate may also be effective and used in various combinations. A crucial part of the treatment of pets with epilepsy is owner education to ensure compliance and successful management.

Feline Epilepsy

Seizures in Feline patients are caused by various onsets. As with dogs, Felines can have reactive, primary (idiopathic) or secondary seizures. Idiopathiseizures are not as common in cats as in dogs however a recent study conducted showed that of 91 feline seizures, 25% were suspected to have Idiopathiepilepsy. In the same group of 91 cats, 50% were secondary seizures and 20% reactive.

Classifications

Idiopathiepilepsy does not have a classification due to the fact there are no known causes of these seizures, however both reactive and symptomatisecondary epilepsy can be placed into classifications.

Symptomatic

Neoplasia

meningiomas, Lymphomas and glial cell brain tumours are the most common cancers in cats and are all common causes of seizures.

Vascular Disease

Vascular disease refers to any condition that effects the flow of blood to the brain and can potentially result in seizure disorders. common vascular diseases in felines include, Feline IschemiEncephalopathy, Polycythemia and Hypertension.

Inflammatory/ Infectious

Any inflammatory or infectious disease that reaches the brain can result in inducing seizures. the most common inflammatory or infectious diseases which cause seizures in cats include, Feline Infectious Peritonitis, Toxoplasmosis and Cryptococcus.

Reactive Seizure Disorders

Many diseases that occur as a result from illness in parts of the body other than the brain can cause felines to have seizures, especially in older cats. Some of the common metabolicauses of seizures in felines include, HepatiEncephalopathy, Renal Encephalopathy, Hypoglycaemia and Hypothyroidism.

Bladder Stone (Animal)

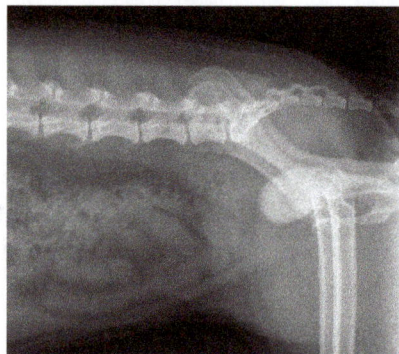

X-ray of a single, large bladder stone in a dog with a bladder located more to the rear than is usual

Bladder stones or uroliths are a common occurrence in animals, especially in domestianimals such as dogs and cats. Occurrence in other species, including tortoises, have been reported as well. The stones form in the urinary bladder in varying size and numbers secondary to infection, dietary influences, and genetics. Stones can form in any part of the urinary tract in dogs and cats, but unlike in humans, stones of the kidney are less common and do not often cause significant disease, although they can contribute to pyelonephritis and chronirenal failure. Types of stones include struvite, calcium oxalate, urate, cystine, calcium phosphate, and silicate. Struvite and calcium oxalate stones are by far the most common.

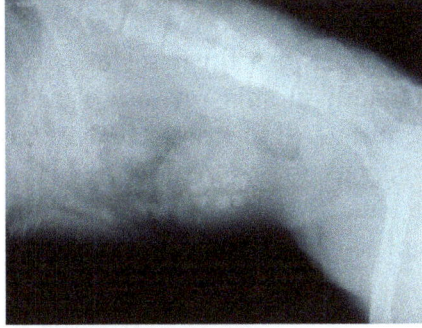

X-ray of bladder stones in a dog

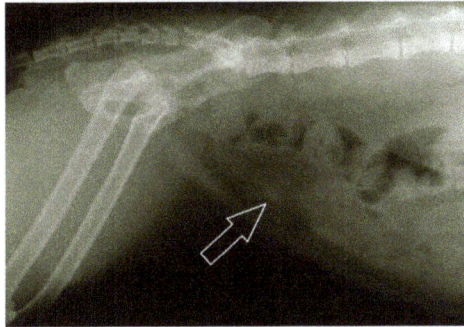

X-ray of a struvite bladder stone in a cat

Signs and Symptoms

Bladder stones may cause blood in the urine (hematuria) (giving the appearance that the animal is urinating blood) but sometimes there may be no signs at all. Painful urination or straining to urinate are other signs. Urinary tract infections are commonly associated with bladder stones. Smaller stones may become lodged in the urethra, especially in male animals, causing urinary tract obstruction and the inability to urinate. This condition causes acute renal failure, hyperkalemia, septicemia, and death within a few days.

Mechanism

Oversaturation of urine with crystals is by the far the biggest factor in 99% of animals in all of Europe. Stone formation. This oversaturation can be caused by increased excretion of crystals by the kidneys, water reabsorption by the renal tubules resulting in concentration of the urine, and changes in urine pH that influence crystallization. Other contributing factors include diet, frequency of urination, genetics, current medications, and the presence of a urinary tract infection.

The stones form around a nidus, which can consist of white blood cells, bacteria, and organimatrix mixed with crystals, or crystals alone. The nidus makes up about two to ten percent of the mass of the stone. It is possible for the nidus to be made of a different type of crystal than the rest of the stone, also known as epitaxial growth.

Diagnosis

When symptoms indicate bladder stones, the first step is usually to take an x-ray. Most types of stones will appear readily in an x-ray, urate and occasionally cystine stones being the most common exceptions. Stones smaller than three millimeters may not be visible. Ultrasonography is also useful for identifying bladder stones. Crystals identified in a urinalysis may help identify the stones, but analysis of the stones is necessary for identification of the complete chemical composition.

Struvite Stones

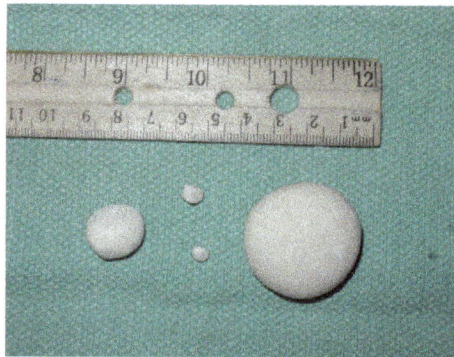

Struvite stones

Struvite stones are also known as magnesium ammonium phosphate stones due to their chemical composition - $MgNH_4PO_4 \cdot 6H_2O$. Often there is a small amount of calcium phosphate present. They form at a neutral to alkaline pH of the urine. Bacterial infections contribute to their formation by increasing the pH of the urine through the urease enzyme in dogs. More than 90 percent of dogs with struvite stones have an associated urease-producing bacterial infection in the urinary tract, but in cats struvite stones usually form in sterile urine. The appearance of the stones vary from large solitary stones to multiple smaller stones. They can assume the shape of the bladder or urethra.

Dissolution of the struvite stones depends on acidification of the urine through diet or urinary acidifiers. Special diets for dissolution also have reduced protein, phosphorus, and magnesium, as well as increased salt to increase water consumption and dilute the urine. The diet needs to be fed exclusively, but it can only be fed for a few months total due to potential side effects. Contraindications to this diet include heart failure, liver failure, kidney failure, pancreatitis, hypertension (high blood pressure), and hypoalbuminemia (low serum albumin). Prevention of struvite stones is with a similar diet with milder restrictions.

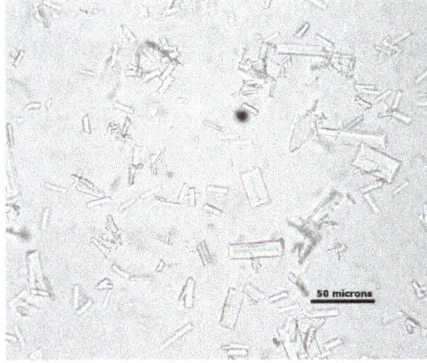
Struvite crystals

Certain dog breeds are predisposed to struvite stones, including Miniature Schnauzers, Bichon Frises, and Cocker Spaniels. They are the most commonly reported bladder stone in female dogs and in ferrets (pregnant ferrets may be especially predisposed).

Calcium Oxalate Stones

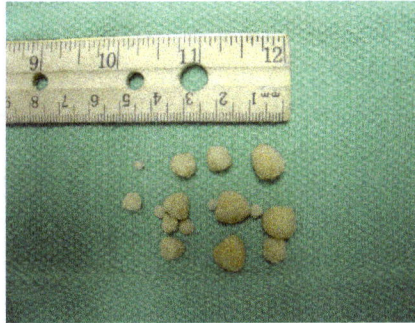
Calcium oxalate stones

Calcium oxalate stones form in an acidito neutral urine. Two types naturally occur, calcium oxalate monohydrate, or whewellite ($CaC_2O_4 \cdot H_2O$), and calcium oxalate dihydrate, or weddellite ($CaC_2O_4 \cdot 2H_2O$). Their appearance can be rough, smooth, spiculated (needle-like), or jackstone. Calcium oxalate stones form more readily in animals with hypercalcaemia, which can caused by Addison's disease or certain types of cancer. Hypercalcaemia results in hypercalciuria, which can also be caused by Cushing's syndrome or hyperparathyroidism.

There is no recommended diet to dissolve calcium oxalate stones. For prevention a diet low in protein and oxalates and high in magnesium, phosphorus, and calcium is recommended. Increased dietary magnesium and phosphorus decreases the amount of calcium in the urine, and increased dietary calcium reduces absorption of oxalates from the intestines. Potassium citrate has been recommended as a preventative for calcium oxalate stone formation because it forms a soluble complex with oxalates and promotes the formation of alkaline urine.

Dog breeds possible prone to calcium oxalate stones include Miniature Schnauzers, Lhasa Apsos, Yorkshire Terriers, Miniature Poodles, Shih Tzus, and Bichon Frises. They are the most common stone in male dogs. Calcium oxalate stones are also common in domestirabbits. Rabbits are prone to hypercalciuria due to intestinal absorption of calcium not being dependent on vitamin D and a high fractional urinary excretion of calcium. The urine will appear thick and creamy or sometimes sandy. Small stones and sand can be removed using urohydropropulsion. Prevention is through reducing calcium intake by feeding more hay and less commercial rabbit pellets, and by not using mineral supplements.

Frequency of Struvite and Calcium Oxalate Stones in Cats

The Minnesota Urolith Center at the University of Minnesota College of Veterinary Medicine has done detailed analysis of uroliths from animals since 1981 and has noted changing trends in feline uroliths. In 1981, struvite stones were the most common type in cats, making up 78 percent of submitted samples, with only 2 percent comprising calcium oxalate stones. In the mid 1980s there was a substantial increase in the number of calcium oxalate samples, and between 1994 and 2002, 55 percent of feline stones were calcium oxalate and 33 percent were struvite. This may have been caused by the use of dissolution diets for struvite stones in cats and modification of other diets to prevent struvite crystal formation. These modifications predisposed to calcium oxalate crystal formation. However, in 2004, struvite stones once again surpassed calcium oxalate stones 44.9 percent to 44.3 percent, and in 2006, 50 percent of stones were struvite and 39 percent were calcium oxalate. This may have been due to the increased use of diets designed to prevent calcium oxalate crystal formation, which because of increased magnesium in the diet and decreased acidity of the urine help promote struvite crystal formation.

Urethral plugs in cats are usually composed of struvite crystals and organimatter.

Urate Stones

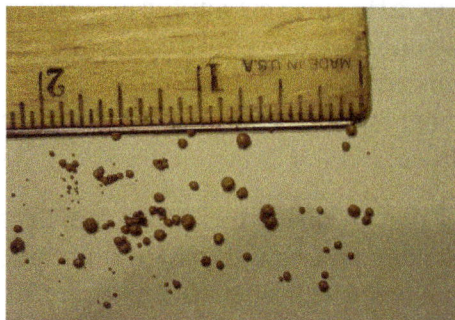

Urate stones

Urate ($C_5H_4N_4O_3$) stones, usually ammonium urate ($NH_4 \cdot C_5H_4N_4O_3$) or sodium urate monohydrate ($Na \cdot C_5H_4N_4O_3 \times H_2O$), form in an acidito neutral urine. They are usually small, yellow-brown, smooth stones. Urate stones form due to an increased excretion of uriacid in the urine. Dalmatians (especially males) and to a lesser extent Bulldogs are genetically predisposed to the formation of urate stones because of an altered metabolism of purines. Dalmatians have a decreased rate of urate hepatitransport, leading to only about 30 to 40 percent conversion of urate to allantoin, compared with greater than 90 percent conversion in other breeds. Dogs with portosystemishunts or endstage liver disease also have increased uriacid excretion in the urine due to reduced conversion of uriacid to allantoin and ammonia to urea. Urate stones make up about six percent of all stones in the cat.

Urate stones can be dissolved using a diet with reduced purines that alkalinizes and dilutes the urine. Allopurinol is used in dogs with altered purine metabolism to prevent the formation of uriacid. Feeding a diet high in purines while simultaneously administering allopurinol can result in the formation of xanthine ($C_5H_4N_4O_2$) stones.

Cystine Stones

Cystine (($SCH_2CHNH_2COOH)_2$) stones form in an acidito neutral urine. They are usually smooth and round. They are caused by increased urine excretion of cystine (a relatively insoluble amino acid) in dogs with a defect in renal tubule reabsorption of cystine. Dietary reduction of protein and alkalinization of the urine may help prevent formation. Medications such as D-penicillamine and 2-MPG contain thiol, which forms a soluble complex with cystine in the urine. Dog breeds possibly predisposed to formation of cystine stones include Bulldogs, Dachshunds, Basset Hounds, Chihuahuas, Yorkshire Terriers, Irish Terriers, and Newfoundlands. In Newfoundlands, cystinuria is inherited as an autosomal recessive trait, but in the other breeds it is a sex linked trait and found primarily in male dogs.

Calcium Phosphate Stones

Calcium phosphate, also known as hydroxyapatite ($Ca_{10}(PO_4)_6(OH)_2$), stones form in neutral to alkaline urine. They are usually smooth and round. Calcium phosphate is usually a component of struvite or calcium oxalate stones and is infrequently a pure stone. They form more readily with hypercalcaemia. Dog breeds possibly predisposed to calcium phosphate stone formation include Yorkshire Terriers, Miniature Schnauzers, and Cocker Spaniels.

Silicate Stones

Silicate (SiO_2) stones form in acidito neutral urine. They are usually jackstone in appearance. There is possibly an increased incidence associated with dogs on diets that have a large amount of corn gluten or soybean hulls. Dog breeds possibly predisposed include German Shepherd Dogs, Golden Retrievers, Labrador Retrievers, and Miniature Schnauzers.

Treatment

Reasons for treatment of bladder stones include recurring symptoms and risk of urinary tract obstruction. Some stones can be dissolved using dietary modifications and/or medications. Small stones in female dogs may possibly be removed by urohydropropulsion, a nonsurgical procedure. Urohydropropulsion is performed under sedation by filling the bladder with saline through a catheter, holding the dog vertically, and squeezing the bladder to expel the stones through the urethra. Bladder stones can be removed surgically by a cystotomy, opening of the bladder. Stones lodged in the urethra can often be flushed into the bladder and removed, but sometimes a urethrotomy is necessary. In male dogs with recurrent urinary tract obstruction a scrotal urethrostomy creates a permanent opening in the urethra proximal to the area where most stones lodge, behind the os penis. In male cats, stones lodge where the urethra narrows in the penis. Recurrent cases can be treated surgically with a perineal urethrostomy, which removes the penis and creates a new opening for the urethra.

To prevent recurrence of stones, special diets can be used for each type of stone. Increasing water consumption by the animal dilutes the urine, which prevents oversaturation of the urine with crystals.

Schistosoma Nasale

Schistosoma nasale is a species of digenetitrematode in the family Schistosomatidae.

Schistosoma nasale was identified in 1933 by Dr. M. A. N. Rao at Madras Veterinary College, Tamil Nadu, India, as a causative agent for "snoring disease" in cattle.

The first intermediate host is a freshwater snail *Indoplanorbis exustus* that may be the sole natural intermediate host for *Schistosoma nasale* (and other two *Schistosoma* species) on the Indian sub-continent. Earlier, other snails are also implicated in transmission of *Schistosoma nasale* as the first intermediate host and they include: *Lymnaea luteola* and *Lymnaea acuminata but experimental work of Dutt and Srivastava (1962) conclusively proved Indoplanorbis exustus as the sole intermediate host of S. nasale.*

Schistosoma nasale inhabits blood vessels of the nasal mucosa and causes "snoring disease" in cattle. and remains symptomless in buffaloes though extruding its eggs in nasal discharge.

The clinical symptoms in cattle include a cauliflower-like growth or granuloma in the nasal cavity, associated with a "snoring" sound and profuse mucopurulent discharge-Template:Rao 1933). In the endemiareas, there are some local cattle which remain negative for S. nasale eggs, others excrete eggs but without exhibiting symptoms, while a large number exhibit symptoms with presence of the eggs in nasal discharge (Agrawal M2012 Schistosomes and schistosomiasis in South Asia. Springer (India) Pvt Ltd, New Delhi). A different form of nasal schistosomiasis where local cattle are negative for Schistosoma nasale but local buffaloes carry it without showing any symptoms has been shown to exist at Jabalpur, Madhya Pradesh; there, cross-bred cattle exhibit snoring disease symptoms with eggs in their nasal discharge (Banerjee PS and Agrawal M1991. Prevalence of Schistosoma nasale Rao 1933 at Jabalpur. *Indian Journal of Animal Sciences* 61:789-791). Anthiomaline was the drug of choice, but this leads to relapse of the symptoms after two months of the treatment. Praziquantel proved better than any other drug but at present it costs Rs 1500 per animal as treatment cost. Recently, Dr. M. C. Agrawal has successfully treated cases of nasal schistosomiasis by administering triclabendazole at a dosage of 20 mg/kg body weight which appears a better alternative looking to cost of the treatment. Nevertheless, there are all chances of killing susceptible blood flukes by these less effective drugs resulting in existence of more resistant schistosome population in future generations causing more problems (Agrawal 2012). schistosoma nasale eggs are boomerang or palaquine shaped.

References

- Carpenter, Kenneth J. (1988). The History of Scurvy and Vitamin C. Cambridge University Press. p. 172. ISBN 0-521-34773-4.

- Fernandez-Armesto, Felipe (2006). Pathfinders: A Global History of Exploration. W.W. Norton & Company. pp. 297–298. ISBN 0-393-06259-7.

- A. S. Turberville (2006). "Johnson's England: An Account of the Life & Manners of His Age". ISBN READ BOOKS. p.53. ISBN 1-4067-2726-1

- Vale and Edwards (2011). Physician to the Fleet; the Life and Times of Thomas Trotter 1760-1832. Woodbridge: The Boydell Press. pp. 29–33. ISBN 978 1 84383 604 9.

- Bown, Stephen R. (2003). Scurvy: How a Surgeon, a Mariner and a Gentleman Solved the Greatest Medical Mystery of the Age of Sail. New York: Viking. ISBN 0-312-31391-8.

- Lamb, Jonathan (2001). Preserving the self in the south seas, 1680–1840. University of Chicago Press. p. 117. ISBN 0-226-46849-6.

- Drymon, M. M. (2008). Disguised As the Devil: How Lyme Disease Created Witches and Changed History. Wythe Avenue Press. p. 114. ISBN 0-615-20061-3.

- Renzaho, Andre M. N. (2016). Globalisation, Migration and Health: Challenges and Opportunities. World Scientific. p. 94. ISBN 9781783268894.

- Hillyer, Elizabeth V.; Quesenberry, Katherin E. (1997). Ferrets, Rabbits, and Rodents: Clinical Medicine and Surgery (1st ed.). W.B. Saunders Company. ISBN 0-7216-4023-0.

- Ettinger, Stephen J.; Feldman, Edward C. (1995). Textbook of Veterinary Internal Medicine (4th ed.). W.B. Saunders Company. ISBN 0-7216-6795-3.

- Morrison, Wallace B. (1998). Cancer in Dogs and Cats (1st ed.). Williams and Wilkins. ISBN 0-683-06105-4.

Veterinary Drugs: A Comprehensive Study

Some of the veterinary drugs mentioned in this section are acepromazine, amitriptyline, boldenone, butorphanol, carprofen, xylazine and neoplasene. Acepromazine is an antipsychotic drug that is used in humans and animals both. This drug is used on animals that are hyperactive or are fractious. The topics discussed in the section are of great importance to broaden the existing knowledge on veterinary drugs.

Acepromazine

Acepromazine or acetylpromazine (more commonly known as ACP, Ace, or by the trade names Atravet or Acezine 2, number depending on mg/ml dose) is a phenothiazine derivative antipsychotic drug. It was used on humans during the 1950s as an antipsychotic, but is now almost exclusively used on animals as a sedative and antiemetic. Its closely related analogue, chlorpromazine, is still used as an antipsychotic in humans. Acepromazine is used primarily as a chemical restraint in hyperactive or fractious animals. However, it does not relieve anxiety, and some believe it may make anxiety worse in the long run if used on an anxious animal (for example, thunderstorm phobias). The standard pharmaceutical preparation, acepromazine maleate, is used in veterinary medicine in dogs, and cats. It is used widely in horses as a pre-anaesthetic sedative and has been shown to reduce anaesthesia related death. However, it should be used with caution (but is not absolutely contraindicated) in stallions due to the risk of paraphimosis and persistent priapism. Its potential for cardiac effects, namely hypotension due to peripheral vasodilation, can be profound and as such is not recommended for use in geriatric or debilitated animals, especially dogs. In these cases it is most often substituted with midazolam or diazepam and left out of the preanesthetic medication altogether.

Pharmacology

The clinical pharmacology of acepromazine is similar to that of other phenothiazine derived anti-psychotic agents. The primary behavioral effects are attributed to its potent antagonism of D2 receptors and, to a lesser degree, the other D2-like receptors. Additional effects are related to its appreciable antagonistic effects on various other receptors, including the α_1 receptors, H_1 receptors, and mACh receptors.

Administration

Canine

When used as a premedication it is commonly administered via the subcutaneous or intramuscular route within the clinic and as single or di-scored unflavoured tablets for oral administration. It is also administered orally prior to travel, veterinary exams, and other predictable situations in which the animal is expected to be exceptionally excited, anxious, uncooperative, or even hostile.

Potential Adverse Effects in Dogs

Literature from the 1950s raised concerns about phenothiazine-induced seizures in human patients. A family of Boxers in the UK were implicated for an increased seizure risk when given acepromazine and it was previously recommended to avoid this medication in this breed. For this reason, caution has typically been advised when contemplating acepromazine use in epileptic canine patients although no veterinary studies have been published until quite recently. The two published veterinary studies have failed to show a positive association between use of acepromazine and seizure activity and show a possible role for acepromazine in seizure control: in a retrospective study at University of Tennessee, acepromazine was administered for tranquilization to 36 dogs with a prior history of seizures and to decrease seizure activity in 11 dogs. No seizures were seen within 16 hours of acepromazine administration in the 36 dogs that received the drug for tranquilization during hospitalization. After acepromazine administration, seizures abated for 1.5 to 8 hours (n=6) or did not recur (n=2) in eight of 10 dogs that were actively seizing. Excitement-induced seizure frequency was reduced for 2 months in one dog. A second retrospective study also concluded that administration of acepromazine to dogs with prior or acute seizure history did not potentiate seizures and there was some trend toward seizure reduction. It should be noted that the original seizure cautions reported in the 1950s were in human patients on relatively high anti-psychotic doses of chlorpromazine while the doses of acepromazine used in the only two published veterinary studies cited above are much lower.

Recently a multi-drug resistance gene (MDR1) has been isolated by researchers at Washington State University College of Veterinary Medicine. Mutations in the gene are more common in certain herding breeds and whippets (although Border Collies are over-represented) as well as many mixed breeds. The mutation causes increased sensitivity to ivermectin and related avermectins, acepromazine, certain opioids and opioid derivatives, as well as vincristine and certain other chemotherapeutics. It is recommended that acepromazine dose be reduced by 25% in heterozygotes and by 30-50% in dogs homozygous for the mutation. Owners may test their dogs via a kit available from WSU and are strongly encouraged to share those results with their veterinarian.

The Boxer is reported to have a breed-related sensitivity to acepromazine. In 1996 a warning was placed in the cardiology section of the Veterinary Information Network

(VIN), a US-based network for practicing veterinarians, entitled "Acepromazine and Boxers." It described several adverse reactions to acepromazine in three Boxers at the University of California at Davis veterinary teaching hospital. The reactions included collapse, respiratory arrest, and profound bradycardia (slow heart rate, less than 60 beats per minute). While there is disagreement among some veterinarians on this point, a number of veterinary publications recommend the drug be avoided in the breed. Individual dogs of any breed can have a profound reaction characterized by hypotension (low blood pressure), especially if there is an underlying heart problem.

Acepromazine should be used with caution in sighthounds.

Equine

Acepromazine can be administered by the intramuscular route, taking effect within 30–45 minutes, or may be given intravenously, taking effect within 15 minutes. Sedation usually lasts for 1–4 hours, although some horses may feel the effects for up to 24 hours. The standard dose is highly variable, depending upon the desired effect following administration. An oral gel formulation is also available (**Sedalin gel**). The dosage by this route is also highly variable, but it is generally accepted that the recommended dose will give moderate sedation in most horses.

In the UK, acepromazine is not authorised for use in horses intended for human consumption. In equine surgery, premedication with acepromazine has been shown to reduce the perianaesthetic mortality rate, although the reasons for this are unclear.

Additionally, acepromazine is used as a vasodilator in the treatment of laminitis, where an oral dose equivalent to "mild sedation" is commonly used, although the dose used is highly dependent on the treating veterinarian. While it is shown to elicit vasodilation in the distal limb, evidence showing its efficacy at increasing perfusion in the laminae is lacking. It is also sometimes used to treat a horse experiencing Equine Exertional Rhabdomyolysis.

Precautions When Using in Horses

Acepromazine is a prohibited class A drug under FEI rules, and its use is prohibited or restricted by many other equestrian organizations. It can be detected in the blood for 72–120 hours, although repeated doses may make it remain present for several months.

Side effects are not common, but the use of acepromazine in stallions should be used with caution (but is not absolutely contraindicated) due to the risk of paraphimosis and priapism.

Acepromazine should not be used in horses dewormed with piperazine. It lowers blood pressure, and should therefore be used with caution in horses that are experiencing anemia, dehydration, shock, or colic.

Feline

Acepromazine is sometimes recommended or prescribed in tiny oral doses to the pet cats of allergy sufferers.

Drug Reaction: MDR1 Gene Deletion

For over 20 years herding dogs have died from negative reactions to acepromazine that were rooted in genetic mutations. This reveals a lack of understanding about acepromazine, and other drugs with potentially toxic side effects. Scientists isolated the problem: the Multi Drug Resistant 1 (MDR1) gene. In addition, more than 30 potentially toxic drugs have been identified, and a lab test has been developed to identify dogs with the abnormal MDR1 gene. Three different factors are now recognized that contribute to drug toxicity especially common in herding dogs: a genetic mutation, drugs that inactivate normal cell pumps, and substances that inactivate cell enzymes so they cannot break down drugs.

In addition to having proteins on the membrane that remove drugs from the cell, most cells have enzymes that break down drugs and inactivate them. Cytochrome P 450 is a family of enzymes that inactivates about 60% of drugs used in pets. One of the CYP 450 family—CYP3A—can be blocked or inactivated by ketoconazole and by grapefruit juice. With CYP3A inactivated, drugs reach toxic concentrations within cells.

Dogs can have both the defective MDR1 gene and have inactivated CYP3A enzymes. These dogs are very likely to develop toxicity with certain drugs.

Breeds with abnormal MDR1 gene

Dogs at risk: Australian Shepherd, Border Collie, Collie, English Shepherd, German Shepherd, Old English Sheepdog, and Sighthounds. Other dogs including mixed breeds, shelties, long haired greyhound may also lack P-glycoprotein transporters.

Drugs that Become Toxic if not Pumped Out by P-glycoproteins

Many different drugs are normally pumped from cells by P-glycoproteins: anticancer drugs, antiparasitics, antibiotics, cardiac drugs, immunosuppressants, opioids, steroid hormones, and miscellaneous drugs. Acepromazine can become toxic in dogs with the MDR1 mutation. The commonly used veterinary antihelmintic ivermectin is another example of a drug which is peripherally acting due to p-glycoprotein.

Drugs like acepromazine can lead to hearing loss and other serious side effects.

Amitriptyline

Amitriptyline, sold under the brand name Elavil among others, is a medicine used to treat a number of mental illnesses. These include major depressive disorder and anx- iety disorder, and less commonly attention deficit hyperactivity disorder and bipolar disorder. Other uses include prevention of migraines, treatment of neuropathic pain such as fibromyalgia and postherpetic neuralgia, and less commonly insomnia. It is in the tricyclic antidepressant (TCA) class and its exact mechanism of action is unclear. Amitriptyline is taken by mouth.

Common side effects include a dry mouth, trouble seeing, low blood pressure on stand- ing, sleepiness, and constipation. Serious side effects may include seizures, an increased risk of suicide in those less than 25 years of age, urinary retention, glaucoma, and a number of heart issues. It should not be taken with MAO inhibitors or the medication cisapride. Amitriptyline may cause problems if taken during pregnancy. Use during breastfeeding appears to be relatively safe.

Amitriptyline was discovered in 1960 and approved by the US Food and Drug Admin- istration (FDA) in 1961. It is on the WHO Model List of Essential Medicines, the most important medications needed in a basic health system. It is available as a generic med- ication. The wholesale cost in the developing world as of 2014 is between 0.01 and 0.04 USD per dose. In the United States it costs about 0.20 USD per dose.

Medical Uses

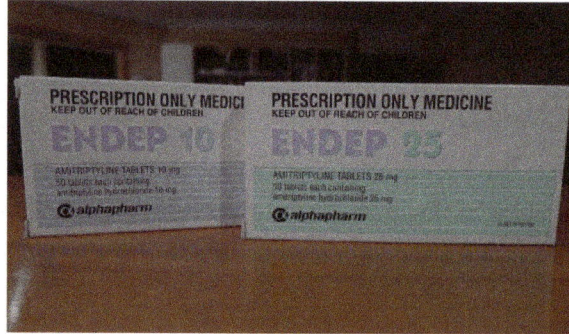

Two boxes of amitriptyline (Endep) in 10- and 25-mg doses

Amitriptyline is used for a number of medical conditions including major depressive disorder (MDD). Some evidence suggests amitriptyline may be more effective than oth- er antidepressants, including selective serotonin reuptake inhibitors (SSRIs), although it is rarely used as a first-line antidepressant due to its higher toxicity in overdose and generally poorer tolerability.

It is TGA-labeled for migraine prevention, also in cases of neuropathic pain disorders, fibromyalgia and nocturnal enuresis. Amitriptyline is a popular off-label treatment for irritable bowel syndrome (IBS), although it is most frequently reserved for severe cases of abdominal pain in patients with IBS because it needs to be taken regularly to work and has a generally poor tolerability profile, although a firm evidence base supports its efficacy in this indication. Amitriptyline can also be used as an anticholinergic drug in the treatment of early-stage Parkinson's disease if depression also needs to be treated. Amitriptyline is the most widely researched agent for prevention of frequent tension headaches.

Investigational Uses

- Eating disorders: The few randomized controlled trials investigating its efficacy in eating disorders have been discouraging.

- Insomnia: As of 2004, amitriptyline was the most commonly prescribed off-label prescription sleep aid in the United States. Owing to the development of tolerance and the potential for adverse effects such as constipation, its use in the elderly for this indication is recommended against.

- Urinary incontinence. An accepted use for amitriptyline in Australia is the treatment of urinary urge incontinence.

- Cyclic vomiting syndrome

- Chronic cough

- Preventive treatment for patients with recurring biliary dyskinesia (sphincter of Oddi dysfunction)

- Attention deficit/hyperactivity disorder (in addition to, or sometimes in place of ADHD stimulant drugs)

- Retching/dry heaving, especially after the anti-reflux procedure Nissen fundoplication

Adverse Effects

Common (≥1% frequency) side effects include dizziness, headache, weight gain, side effects common to anticholinergics, but more such effects than other TCAs, cognitive effects such as delirium and confusion, mood disturbances such as anxiety and agitation, cardiovascular side effects such as orthostatic hypotension and sinus tachycardia, sexual side effects such as loss of libido and impotence, and sleep disturbances such as drowsiness, insomnia and nightmares.

Contraindications

The known contraindications of amitriptyline are:

- Hypersensitivity to tricyclic antidepressants or to any of its excipients

- History of myocardial infarction

- History of arrhythmias, particularly heart block to any degree

- Congestive heart failure

- Coronary artery insufficiency

- Mania

- Severe liver disease

- Children under 7 years

- Breast feeding

- Patients who are taking monoamine oxidase inhibitors (MAOIs) or have taken them within the last 14 days.

Interactions

Amitriptyline is known to interact with:

- Monoamine oxidase inhibitors as it can potentially induce a serotonin syndrome

- CYP2D6 inhibitors and substrates such as fluoxetine due to the potential for an increase in plasma concentrations of the drug to be seen

- Guanethidine as it can reduce the antihypertensive effects of this drug

- Anticholinergic agents such as benztropine, hyoscine (scopolamine) and atropine, because the two might exacerbate each other's anticholinergic effects, including paralytic ileus and tachycardia

- Antipsychotics due to the potential for them to exacerbate the sedative, anticholinergic, epileptogenic and pyrexic (fever-promoting) effects. Also increases the risk of neuroleptic malignant syndrome

- Cimetidine due to the potential for it to interfere with hepatic metabolism of amitriptyline and hence increasing steady-state concentrations of the drug

- Disulfiram due to the potential for the development of delirium

- ECT may increase the risks associated with this treatment

- Antithyroid medications may increase the risk of agranulocytosis

- Thyroid hormones have a potential for increased adverse effects such as CNS stimulation and arrhythmias.

- Analgesics, such as tramadol, due to the potential for an increase in seizure risk

- Medications subject to gastric inactivation (e.g. levodopa) due to the potential for amitriptyline to delay gastric emptying and reduce intestinal motility

- Medications subject to increased absorption given more time in the small intestine (e.g. anticoagulants)
- Serotoninergic agents such as the SSRIs and triptans due to the potential for serotonin syndrome.

Overdose

The symptoms and the treatment of an overdose are largely the same as for the other TCAs, including the presentation of serotonin syndrome and adverse cardiac effects. The British National Formulary notes that amitriptyline can be particularly dangerous in overdose, thus it and other tricyclic antidepressants are no longer recommended as first-line therapy for depression. Alternative agents, SSRIs and SNRIs, are safer in overdose, though they are no more efficacious than TCAs. English folk singer Nick Drake died from an overdose of Tryptizol in 1974.

The possible symptoms of amitriptyline overdose include:

- Drowsiness
- Hypothermia (low body temperature)
- Tachycardia (high heart rate)
- Other arrhythmic abnormalities, such as bundle branch block
- ECG evidence of impaired conduction
- Congestive heart failure
- Dilated pupils
- Convulsions (e.g. seizures, myoclonus)
- Severe hypotension (very low blood pressure)
- Stupor
- Coma
- Death
- Polyradiculoneuropathy
- Changes in the electrocardiogram, particularly in QRS axis or width
- Agitation
- Hyperactive reflexes
- Muscle rigidity
- Vomiting

The treatment of overdose is mostly supportive as no specific antidote for amitriptyline overdose is available. Activated charcoal may reduce absorption if given within 1–2 hours of ingestion. If the affected person is unconscious or has an impaired gag reflex, a nasogastric tube may be used to deliver the activated charcoal into the stomach. ECG monitoring for cardiac conduction abnormalities is essential and if one is found close monitoring of cardiac function is advised. Body temperature should be regulated with measures such as heating blankets if necessary. Likewise, cardiac arrhythmias can be treated with propranolol and should heart failure occur, digitalis may be used. Cardiac monitoring is advised for at least five days after the overdose. Amitriptyline increases the CNS depressant action, but not the anticonvulsant action of barbiturates; therefore, an inhalation anaesthetic or diazepam is recommended for control of convulsions. Dialysis is of no use due to the high degree of protein binding with amitriptyline.

Mechanism of Action

Receptor	K_i [nM] (amitriptyline)	K_i [nM] (nortriptyline)
SERT	3.13	16.5
NET	22.4	4.37
DAT	5380	3100
5-HT$_{1A}$	450	294
5-HT$_{1B}$	840	-
5-HT$_{2A}$	4.3	5
5-HT$_{2C}$	6.15	8.5
5-HT$_6$	103	148
5-HT$_7$	114	-
H$_1$	1.1	15.1
H$_3$	1000	-
H$_4$	33.6	-
M$_1$	12.9	40
M$_2$	11.8	110
M$_3$	25.9	50
M$_4$	7.2	84
M$_5$	19.9	97
α_1	24	55
α_2	690	2030
D$_1$	89	-
D$_2$	1460	2570
D$_3$	206	-
D$_5$	170	-
σ	300	2000

Amitriptyline acts primarily as a serotonin-norepinephrine reuptake inhibitor, with strong actions on the serotonin transporter and moderate effects on the norepinephrine transporter. It has negligible influence on the dopamine transporter and therefore does not affect dopamine reuptake, being nearly 1,000 times weaker on it than on serotonin. It is metabolised to nortriptyline—a more potent and selective norepinephrine reuptake inhibitor—which may complement its effects on norepinephrine reuptake.

Amitriptyline additionally functions as a $5\text{-}HT_{2A}$, $5\text{-}HT_{2C}$, $5\text{-}HT_3$, $5\text{-}HT_6$, $5\text{-}HT_7$, α_1-adrenergic, H_1, H_2, H_4, and mACh receptor antagonist, and σ_1 receptor agonist. It has also been shown to be a relatively weak NMDA receptor negative allosteric modulator at the same binding site as phencyclidine. Amitriptyline inhibits sodium channels, L-type calcium channels, and $K_v1.1$, $K_v7.2$, and $K_v7.3$ voltage-gated potassium channels, and therefore acts as a sodium, calcium, and potassium channel blocker as well.

Recently, amitriptyline has been demonstrated to act as an agonist of the TrkA and TrkB receptors. It promotes the heterodimerization of these proteins in the absence of NGF and has potent neurotrophic activity both *in-vivo* and *in-vitro* in mouse models. These are the same receptors BDNF activates, an endogenous neurotrophin with powerful antidepressant effects, and as such this property may contribute significantly to its therapeutic efficacy against depression. Amitriptyline also acts as a functional inhibitor of acid sphingomyelinase.

Pharmacokinetics

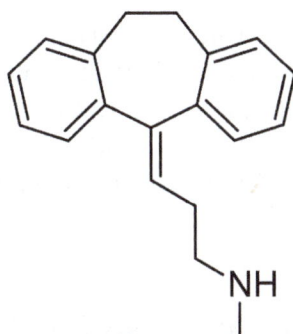

Nortriptyline, amitriptyline's chief active metabolite

Amitriptyline is a highly lipophilic molecule having a log P (octanol/water, pH 7.4) of 3.0, while the intrinsic log P of the free base was reported as 5.04.

Amitriptyline is readily absorbed from the gastrointestinal tract and is extensively metabolised on first pass through the liver. It is metabolised mostly by CYP2D6, CYP3A4, and CYP2C19-mediated N-demethylation into nortriptyline, which is another tricyclic antidepressant in its own right. It is 96% bound to plasma proteins, nortriptyline is 93-95% bound to plasma proteins. It is mostly excreted in the urine (around 30–50%) as metabolites either free or as glucuronide and sulfate conjugates. Small amounts are also excreted in feces.

Pharmacogenetics

Since amitriptyline is primarily metabolized by CYP2D6 and CYP2C19, genetic variations within the genes coding for these enzymes can affect its metabolism, leading to changes in the concentrations of the drug in the body. Increased concentrations of amitriptyline may increase the risk for side effects, including anticholinergic and nervous system adverse effects, while decreased concentrations may reduce the drug's efficacy.

Individuals can be categorized into different types of CYP2D6 or CYP2C19 metabolizers depending on which genetic variations they carry. These metabolizer types include poor, intermediate, extensive, and ultrarapid metabolizers. Most individuals (about 77-92%) are extensive metabolizers, and have "normal" metabolism of amitriptyline. Poor and intermediate metabolizers have reduced metabolism of the drug as compared to extensive metabolizers; patients with these metabolizer types may have an increased probability of experiencing side effects. Ultrarapid metabolizers use amitriptyline much faster than extensive metabolizers; patients with this metabolizer type may have a greater chance of experiencing pharmacological failure.

The Clinical Pharmacogenetics Implementation Consortium recommends avoiding amitriptyline in patients who are CYP2D6 ultrarapid or poor metabolizers, due to the risk for a lack of efficacy and side effects, respectively. The consortium also recommends considering an alternative drug not metabolized by CYP2C19 in patients who are CYP2C19 ultrarapid metabolizers. A reduction in starting dose is recommended for patients who are CYP2D6 intermediate metabolizers and CYP2C19 poor metabolizers. If use of amitriptyline is warranted, therapeutic drug monitoring is recommended to guide dose adjustments. The Dutch Pharmacogenetics Working Group also recommends selecting an alternative drug or monitoring plasma concentrations of amitriptyline in patients who are CYP2D6 poor or ultrarapid metabolizers, and selecting an alternative drug or reducing initial dose in patients who are CYP2D6 intermediate metabolizers.

Brand Names

Brand names include (just including those used in English-speaking countries with † to indicate discontinued brands):

- Amirol (NZ)
- Amit (IN)
- Amitone (IN)
- Amitor (IN)
- Amitrip (AU,† IN, NZ)
- Amitriptyline (UK)

- Amitriptyline Hydrochloride (UK)
- Amitriptyline Hydrochloride Caraco (US)
- Amitriptyline Hydrochloride Mutual (US)
- Amitriptyline Hydrochloride Mylan (US)
- Amitriptyline Hydrochloride Sandoz (US)
- Amitriptyline Hydrochloride Vintage (US)
- Amitrol† (AU)
- Amrea (IN)
- Amypres (IN)
- Apo-Amitriptyline (CA, HK, SG)
- Crypton (IN)
- Elavil (CA, UK†, US†)
- Eliwel (IN)
- Endep (AU, HK]]† , ZA†, US†)
- Enovil† (US)
- Gentrip (IN)
- Kamitrin (IN)
- Laroxyl(FR)
- Latilin (IN)
- Levate (US)
- Maxitrip (IN)
- Mitryp (IN)
- Mitryp-10 (IN)
- Odep (IN)
- Redomex (BE)
- Qualitriptine (HK)

- Sandoz Amitriptyline (ZA)

- Saroten (CH)

- Sarotena (IN)

- Tadamit (IN)

- Trepiline (ZA)

- Tripta (SG) (TH)

- Triptaz (IN)

- Tryptanol (ZA)

- Tryptizol (Spain)

- Triptyl (FI)

- Tryptomer (IN)

Boldenone

Boldenone (INN, BAN), also known as Δ^1-testosterone, 1-dehydrotestosterone, or androsta-1,4-dien-3-one-17β-ol, is a synthetic anabolic-androgenic steroid (AAS) and the 1(2)-dehydrogenated analogue of testosterone. Boldenone itself has never been marketed; as a pharmaceutical drug, it is used as boldenone undecylenate, the undecylenate ester.

Effects and Side-effects

The activity of boldenone is mainly anabolic, with a low androgenic potency. Boldenone will increase nitrogen retention, protein synthesis, increases appetite and stimulates the release of erythropoietin in the kidneys. Boldenone was synthesized in an attempt to create a long-acting injectable methandrostenolone (Dianabol), for androgen deficiency disorders. Boldenone acts similar to methandrostenolone with fewer adverse androgenic effects.Although commonly compared to nandrolone, boldenone lacks progesterone receptor interaction and all the associated progestogenic side effects.

Use in Sports

Baseball

Boldenone is among the substances banned by Major League Baseball, as well as most other major athletic organizations. Los Angeles Angels minor league outfielder Reynaldo Ruiz in September 2010 and Philadelphia Phillies minor league pitcher San Lazaro Solano in January 2011 each received a 50-game suspension for the 2011 season as a result of testing positive for a metabolite of boldenone. Jenrry Mejia, formerly of the New York Mets, was suspended in July 2015 when he tested positive for boldenone and stanozolol, and in February 2016 he again tested positive for boldenone; this marked Mejia's third positive test for a performance-enhancing drug, for which he received the first PED-related lifetime ban in MLB history. Abraham Almonte was suspended for 80 games before the 2016 season after testing positive for boldenone.

Mixed Martial Arts

Stephan Bonnar and Josh Barnett, mixed martial arts (MMA) fighters from the UFC and PRIDE Fighting Championships, have also tested positive for the banned substance. After the World Extreme Cagefighting show on January 20, 2006 Muay Thai turned MMA fighter Kit Cope also tested positive for boldenone. Following the Strikeforce card on June 22, 2007 former PRIDE and UFC fighter Phil Baroni tested positive for boldenone, as well as stanozolol. At a K-1 WGP event in Las Vegas on August 17, 2007 two fighters, Rickard Nordstrand and Zabit Samedov, both tested positive for boldenone. Alexandre Franca Nogueira tested positive for boldenone in July 2008.

Antonio Silva tested positive for boldenone after his July 26, 2008 fight against Justin Eilers in the EliteXC promotion. Silva was suspended by the California State Athletic Commission for a year and fined $2500.

Australian Football League

Justin Charles, a former minor league baseball player with the Florida Marlins, of Richmond FC tested positive for the substance in 1997 and was suspended for 16 matches.

Major League Soccer

Jon Conway (goal keeper) and Jeff Parke (defender) of the New York Red Bulls both tested positive for the substance in 2008 and were suspended 10 games and fined 10% of their annual income. They are also the first to abuse MLS drug policy.

Horse Racing

Leading horse trainer Gai Waterhouse was fined $10,000 after being found guilty on the 15th of May 2008 of presenting a horse to the races with a prohibited substance in its system. Her horse Perfectly Poised was found to have traces of the banned substance boldenone in its system after finishing second at Canterbury in April 2007.

Butorphanol

Butorphanol (AAN, BAN, INN and USAN) is a morphinan-type synthetic opioid analgesic developed by Bristol-Myers. Brand name Stadol was recently discontinued by the manufacturer. It is now only available in its generic formulations, manufactured by Novex, Mylan, Apotex and Ben Venue Laboratories. Butorphanol is most closely structurally related to levorphanol. Butorphanol is available as the tartrate salt in injectable, tablet, and intranasal spray formulations. The tablet form is only used in dogs and cats due to low bioavailability in humans.

Butorphanol is listed under the Single Convention on Narcotic Drugs 1961 and in the United States is a Schedule IV Narcotic controlled substance with a DEA ACSCN of 9720; being in Schedule IV it is not subject to annual aggregate manufacturing quotas. The free base conversion ratio of the hydrochloride is 0.69. Butorphanol was originally in Schedule II and at one point it was decontrolled. Butorphanol derived from thebaine was scheduled separately as Schedule II, then decontrolled on 14. July 1992 and put in Schedule IV on 31. October 1997.

Mechanism of Action

Butorphanol exhibits partial agonist and antagonist activity at the μ-opioid receptor, as well as partial agonist activity at the κ-opioid receptor (K_i = 2.5 nM; EC_{50} = 57 nM; E_{max} = 57%). Stimulation of these receptors on central nervous system neurons causes an intracellular inhibition of adenylate cyclase, closing of influx membrane calcium channels, and opening of membrane potassium channels. This leads to hyperpolarization of the cell membrane potential and suppression of action potential transmission of ascending pain pathways. Because of its κ-agonist activity, at analgesic doses butorphanol increases pulmonary arterial pressure and cardiac work. Additionally, κ-agonism can cause dysphoria at therapeutic or supertherapeutic doses; this gives butorphanol a lower potential for abuse than other opioid drugs.

Place in Therapy

The most common indication for butorphanol is management of migraine using the intranasal spray formulation. It may also be used parenterally for management of moderate-to-severe pain, as a supplement for balanced general anesthesia, and management of pain during labor. Butorphanol is also quite effective at reducing post-operative shivering (owing to its Kappa agonist activity). Butorphanol is more effective in reducing pain in women than in men.

In veterinary use, butorphanol ("Torbugesic") is widely used as a sedative and analgesic in dogs, cats and horses. For sedation, it may be combined with tranquilizers such as alpha-2 agonists (medetomidine (Domitor)), benzodiazepines, or phenothiazines (acepromazine) in dogs, cats and exotic animals. It is frequently combined with xylazine or detomidine (Dormosedan etc.) in horses.

Adverse Effects

As with other opioid analgesics, central nervous system effects (such as sedation, confusion, and dizziness) are considerations with butorphanol. Nausea and vomiting are common. Less common are the gastrointestinal effects of other opioids (mostly constipation). Another side effect experienced by people taking the medication is increased perspiration.

Proprietary Preparations

Butorphanol is available in the U.S. as a generic drug; it is available in various nations under one of any number of trade names, including Moradol and Beforal (Brand name Stadol no longer available in the US); veterinary trade names include Butorphic, Dolorex, Morphasol, Torbugesic, and Torbutrol.

Use in Horses

Butorphanol is a commonly used narcotic for pain relief in horses. It is administered either IM or IV, with its analgestic properties beginning to take effect about 15 minutes after injection and lasting 4 hours. It is also commonly paired with sedatives, such as xylazine and detomidine, to make the horse easier to handle during veterinary procedures.

Side Effects, Overdose, and Precautions

Side effects specific to horses include sedation, CNS excitement (displayed by head pressing or tossing). Overdosing may result in seizures, falling, salivation, constipation, and muscle twitching. If an overdose occurs, a narcotic antagonist, such as naloxone, may be given. Caution should be used if Butorphanol is administered in addition to other narcotics, sedatives, depressants, or antihistamines as it will cause an additive effect.

Butorphanol can cross the placenta, and it will be present in the milk of lactating mares who are given the drug.

The drug is also prohibited for use in competition by most equestrian organizations, including the FEI, which considers it a class A drug.

In addition to horses, butorphanol with or without acepromazine is frequently used in veterinary settings for post-operative and accident-related pain in small mammals such as dogs, cats, ferrets, coatis, raccoons, mongooses, various marsupials, some rodents and perhaps some larger birds both in the operating suite and as a regular prescription medication for home use for management of moderate to severe pain. The efficacy of opioids (as well as other drugs that slow down the system like anaesthetics) in treating reptiles is a question about which there is currently not a lot of data.

Carprofen

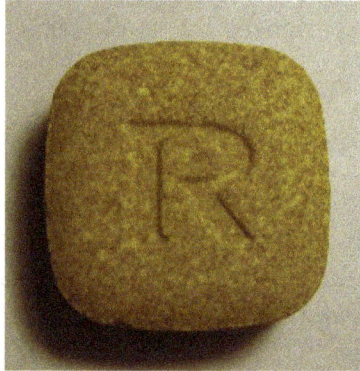

A 100 mg Rimadyl pill approximately 19 mm (0.75 in) wide and 8.6 mm (0.34 in) thick, sold in the United States

Carprofen, marketed under many brand names worldwide, is a non-steroidal anti-inflammatory drug that veterinarians prescribe as a supportive treatment for various conditions in animals. It provides day-to-day treatment for pain and inflammation from various kinds of joint pain as well as post-operative pain. Carprofen reduces inflammation by inhibition of COX-1 and COX-2; its specificity for COX-2 varies from species to species.

Health Issues

Most dogs respond well to carprofen use, but like all non-steroidal anti-inflammatory (NSAID) medications used in humans and animals, it is capable of causing gastrointestinal, liver and kidney problems in some patients.

After introduction, significant anecdotal reports of sudden animal deaths from its use arose. To date, the FDA has received more than 6,000 adverse reaction reports about the drug (manufactured by Pfizer). As a result, the FDA requested that Pfizer advise consumers in their advertising that death is a possible side effect. Pfizer refused and pulled their advertising; however, they now include death as a possible side effect on the drug label. Plans call for a "Dear Doctor" letter to advise veterinarians, and a safety sheet attached to pill packages.

Pfizer acknowledges a problem with some dog owners, especially a consumer group that mounted a campaign dubbed BARKS, for Be Aware of Rimadyl's Known Side-effects—which include loss of appetite, wobbling, vomiting, seizures, and severe liver malfunction. Reports say the drug company has contacted pet owners who told their stories on the Internet, offering to pay medical and diagnostic expenses for dogs that carprofen may have harmed.

Symptoms to watch for include:

- Loss of appetite

- Vomiting

- Diarrhea

- Increase in thirst

- Increase in urination

- Fatigue and/or Lethargy

- Loss of coordination

- Seizures

Other symptoms worth discussing with a vet include excessive drinking or urination, blood or dark tar-like material in urine or stools, jaundice (yellowing of eyes), and unusual lethargy.

Other side effects of Rimadyl include:

- Black, tarry stools or flecks of blood in the vomit

- Drowsiness

- Staggering, stumbling, weakness or partial paralysis, full paralysis, dizziness, loss of balance.

- Change in urination habits (frequency, color, or smell)

- Change in skin (redness, scabs, or scratching)

- Change in behavior (such as decreased or increased activity level, seizure or aggression).

Excess use of Rimadyl can lead to gastritis and ulcer formation. It is also believed that in some breeds of dogs it may induce kidney and liver damage.

Carprofen should not be administered to animals that are also being given steroids (one of the primary risks of this combination being that it can cause ulcers in the stomach). In dogs, it is recommended that the dog be taken off carprofen for three full days before ingesting a steroid (such as prednisolone).

According to the official Rimadyl website, the drug should not be given at the same time with other types of medications such as other NSAIDs (aspirin, etodolac, deracoxib, meloxicam, tepoxalin) or steroids such as dexamethasone, triamcinolone, cortisone or prednisone. However, dog owners whose pets have been administered Rimadyl and have experienced side effects are highly recommended to contact a veterinarian as soon as they appear and to stop the therapy.

Also, Rimadyl must be used with caution within the supervision of a veterinarian in dogs with liver or kidney disease, dehydration, bleeding deficits, or other health problems. Rimadyl is not recommended for use in dogs with bleeding disorders (such as Von Willebrand's disease), as safety has not been established in dogs with these disorders. Also, it has not yet been established whether Rimadyl can be safely used in pregnant dogs, dogs used for breeding purposes, or in lactating female dogs.

Several laboratory studies and clinical trials have been conducted to establish the safety of using Rimadyl. Clinical studies were conducted in nearly 300 dogs, coming from different breeds. These dogs have been treated with Rimadyl at the recommended dose for 2 weeks. According to these studies, the drug was clinically well tolerated and dogs treated with Rimadyl did not have a greater incidence of adverse reactions when compared to the control group.

There are however a number of factors that may contribute to the high incidence of adverse reports received for Rimadyl by the Center for Veterinary Medicine in the late 1990s. These include:

- The type of drug;

- Wide use;

- Duration of use. While the side effects from Rimadyl are known to occur within a short period of time after administration, it is believed that long-term use may actually result in a higher risk for adverse reactions;

- Senior dog use. Older dogs are generally more prone to side effects caused by carprofen.

Human Use

Carprofen was used in humans for almost 10 years, starting in 1988. It was used for the same conditions as in dogs, viz., joint pain and inflammation. The human body accepted the drug well and side effects tended to be mild, usually consisting of nausea or gastro-intestinal pain and diarrhea. For human use, Rimadyl was available only by prescription in 150 to 600 mg doses. Dosage over 250 mg was only for relieving pain after severe trauma, such as post-surgery inflammation. 150 mg doses were commonly used to relieve the pain of arthritis, while 200 mg doses were commonly prescribed in cases of severe arthritis or severe inflammation pain. The drug was taken orally. Pfizer voluntarily pulled it from the market for human use on commercial grounds.

Equine Use

Carprofen is given intravenously to horses at a dose of 0.7 mg/kg once daily. A single dose has been shown to reduce prostaglandin E2 production and inflammatory exudate for up to 15 hours, although there was less effect on eicosanoid production when compared to the effects produced by NSAIDs such as phenylbutazone or flunixin. Prostaglandin E2 and inflammatory exudate are better reduced at a dose of 4 mg/kg IV, with the added benefit of inhibition of leukotriene B4. Carprofen can also be given orally, but intramuscular use may produce muscle damage.

Brands and Dosage Forms

It is marketed under many brand names including:

- Carprieve LA (veterinary use) byNorbrook
- Carprocow (veterinary use) by Norbrook
- Carprodolor (veterinary use) by Le Vet and Virbac
- Carprodyl (veterinary use) by Ceva
- Carprofelican (veterinary use) by Le Vet
- Carprofen (veterinary use) by Apex
- Carprofen Krka (veterinary use) by Krka
- Carprogesic (veterinary use) by Norbrook and Zoetis
- Carprosol (veterinary use) by CP Pharma and Norbrook
- Carprotab (veterinary use) by CPPharma
- Carprox (veterinary use) by Krka and Virbac
- Comforion (veterinary use) by Orion
- Dolagis (veterinary use) by Albrecht, Ati, Scanvet, and Sogeval
- Dolocarp (veterinary use) by Animalcare, Animedic, aniMedica, and Gräub
- Dolox (veterinary use) by Faunapharma
- Eurofen (veterinary use) by Eurovet
- Kelaprofen (veterinary use) by Kela

- Norocarp (veterinary use) by Axience, Norbrook, N-vet, Ufamed, Vetoquinol, and Vet Medic

- Norodyl (veterinary use) by Norbrook

- Paracarp (veterinary use) by IDT

- Prolet (veterinary use) by Jurox

- Reproval (veterinary use) by Norbrook

- Rimadyl (veterinary use) by Orionm Pfizer, Austria; Pfizer, Putney, Wirtz, and Zoetis

- Rimifin (veterinary use) by Albrecht, Chanelle, Eurovet, and Vetoquinol

- Rofeniflex (veterinary use) by Chanelle

- Rycarfa (veterinary use) by Krka

- Scanodyl (veterinary use) by Scan Vet

- Tergive (veterinary use) by Parnell

- Xelcor (veterinary use) by Bayer

Veterinary dosage forms include 25 mg, 75 mg, and 100 mg tablets, and 50 mg per mL injectable form.

Cyproheptadine

Cyproheptadine sold under the brand name Periactin or Peritol, is a first-generation antihistamine with additional anticholinergic, antiserotonergic, and local anesthetic properties.

Medical Uses

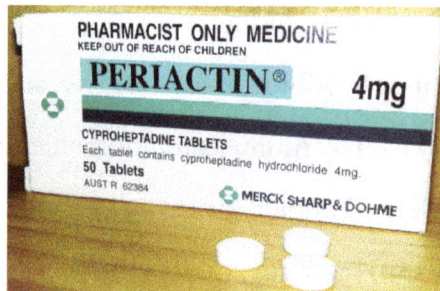

Periactin (cyproheptadine) 4 mg tablets

- Cyproheptadine is used to treat allergic reactions (specifically hay fever). It is also used to treat vasomotor mucosal edema, including vasomotor rhinitis and edema of the throat.

- It has shown effectiveness in the treatment of nightmares, including those related to post-traumatic stress disorder.

- It has been used in the management of moderate to severe cases of serotonin syndrome, a complex of symptoms associated with the use of serotonergic drugs, such as selective serotonin reuptake inhibitors and monoamine oxidase inhibitors), and in cases of high levels of serotonin in the blood resulting from a serotonin-producing carcinoid tumor.

- It can also be used as a preventive measure against migraine in children and adolescents. In Australia this is the only indication for which cyproheptadine is subsidised by the PBS.

- It can relieve SSRI-induced sexual dysfunction and drug-induced hyperhidrosis (excessive sweating).

- It is also used in the treatment of cyclical vomiting syndrome

- Use of the drug can stimulate the appetite and may lead to weight gain, which is helpful for underweight people.

- According to a small study, cyproheptadine hydrochloride has been found to improve sleep, calmness, and mood and energy levels, and to improve both negative and (sometimes even) positive psychotic symptoms in a subgroup of chronic schizophrenics who did not respond (either completely or sufficiently) to other therapies.

- Cyproheptadine may improve akathisia in patients on antipsychotic medications.

- In clinical trials in which cyproheptadine was used as an adjunct to antipsychotic treatment for patients with schizophrenia, an improvement in negative symptoms was seen.

Adverse Effects

Adverse Effects Include

- Sedation and sleepiness (often transient)

- Dizziness

- Disturbed coordination

- Confusion
- Restlessness
- Excitation
- Nervousness
- Tremor
- Irritability
- Insomnia
- Paresthesias
- Neuritis
- Convulsions
- Euphoria
- Hallucinations
- Hysteria
- Faintness
- Allergic manifestation of rash and edema
- Diphoresis
- Urticaria
- Photosensitivity
- Acute labyrinthitis
- Diplopia (seeing double)
- Vertigo
- Tinnitus
- Hypotension (low blood pressure)
- Palpitation
- Extrasystoles
- Anaphylactic shock

- Hemolytic anemia

- Blood dyscrasias such as leukopenia, agranulocytosis and thrombocytopenia

- Cholestasis

- Hepatic (liver) side effects such as:

  - Hepatitis

  - Jaundice

  - Hepatic failure

  - Hepatic function abnormality

- Epigastric distress

- Anorexia

- Nausea

- Vomiting

- Diarrhea

- Anticholinergic side effects such as:

  - Blurred vision

  - Constipation

  - Xerostomia (dry mouth)

  - Tachycardia (high heart rate)

  - Urinary retention

  - Difficulty passing urine

  - Nasal congestion

  - Nasal or throat dryness

- Urinary frequency

- Early menses

- Thickening of bronchial secretions

- Tightness of chest and wheezing

- Fatigue

- Chills
- Headache
- Erectle Dysfunction
- Increased appetite
- Weight gain

Research has shown a suppression of growth hormone with doses of 8–12 mg per day taken for 5 days.

Overdose

Gastric decontamination measures such as activated charcoal are sometimes recommended in cases of overdose. The symptoms are usually indicative of CNS depression (or conversely CNS stimulation in some) and excess anticholinergic side effects. The LD_{50} in mice is 123 mg/kg and 295 mg/kg in rats.

Pharmacology

Cyproheptadine is known to be an antagonist (or inverse agonist depending on the site in question) of the receptors listed in the table below.

Receptor/Transporter Protein	Binding affinity (K_i[nM]) towards cloned human receptors unless otherwise specified
SERT	4100 (RC)
NET	290 (RC)
5-HT_{1A}	59
5-HT_{2A}	1.67
5-HT_{2B}	1.54
5-HT_{2C}	2.23
5-HT_{3}	228 (MN)
5-HT_{6}	142
5-HT_{7}	123.01
M_1	12
M_2	7
M_3	12
M_4	8
M_5	11.8
D_1	117
D_2	112
D_3	8
H_1	0.06

H$_3$	>10000
H$_4$	201.5

Acronyms used:RC - Cloned rat receptor.MN - Mouse NG108-15 receptor.

Pharmacokinetics

Cyproheptadine is well-absorbed following oral ingestion, with peak plasma levels occurring after 1–3 hours. Its half-life when taken orally is approximately 8 hours.

Veterinary Use

Cyproheptadine is used in cats as an appetite stimulant and as an adjunct in the treatment of asthma. Possible adverse effects include excitement and aggressive behavior. The elimination half-life of cyproheptadine in cats is 12 hours.

Cyproheptadine has been used successfully in treatment of pituitary pars intermedia dysfunction in horses.

Pentobarbital

Pentobarbital (US English) or pentobarbitone (UK English) is a short-acting barbiturate. Pentobarbital can occur as both a free acid and as salts of elements such as sodium and calcium. The free acid is only slightly soluble in water and ethanol.

One brand name for this drug is Nembutal, coined by John S. Lundy, who started using it in 1930, from the structural formula of the sodium salt—Na (sodium) + ethyl + methyl + butyl + al (common suffix for barbiturates). Nembutal is trademarked and manufactured by the Danish pharmaceutical company Lundbeck, and is the only injectable form of pentobarbital approved for sale in the United States.

In high doses, pentobarbital causes death by respiratory arrest. In the United States, the drug has been used for executions of convicted criminals. Lundbeck (one of many manufacturers) does not permit its sale to prisons or corrections departments to carry out the death penalty.

Uses

Medical

Typical applications for pentobarbital are sedative, hypnotic for short term, preanesthetic and control of convulsions in emergencies.

It is also used as a veterinary anesthetic agent.

Pentobarbital also has an application in reducing intracranial pressure in Reye's syndrome, traumatic brain injury and induction of coma in cerebral ischemia patients. Pentobarbital-induced coma has been advocated in patients with acute liver failure refractory to mannitol.

Euthanasia

Pentobarbital can induce death when used in high doses. It is used for euthanasia for humans as well as nonhumans. It is also used by itself, or in combination with complementary agents such as phenytoin, in commercial animal euthanasia injectable solutions.

In the Netherlands, the standard protocol for physician-assisted suicide is intravenously induced thiopental anesthesia, followed by bromide of alcuronium- or pancuronium-induced respiratory arrest. A concentrated oral solution of 100 mL containing 9 grams of pentobarbital sodium along with sugar syrup in a 20% ethanol solution is a standard solution used for self-administration by patient.

The oral dosage of pentobarbital indicated for physician-assisted death in the United States states of Oregon, Washington, Vermont, and California (as of January, 2016) is typically 10 g in liquid form. This is considerably higher than the dose for the management of status epilepticus.

Capital Punishment

Pentobarbital has been used or considered as a substitute for other drugs traditionally used in the United States for execution when they are in short supply. Such use however is illegal under Danish law, and when this was discovered, after public outcry in Danish media, Lundbeck, the owner of the drug, stopped selling it to US States that practice death penalty. US distributors of the drug are forbidden by the owner to sell it to any customers, such as several state authorities, that practice or participate in executions of humans.

Texas began using pentobarbital for executing death row inmates by lethal injection on July 18, 2012. The use of pentobarbital has been considered by several states, including Ohio, Arizona, Idaho and Washington; those states made the decision to switch following shortages of pancuronium bromide, a muscle relaxant previously used as one component in a three-drug cocktail.

In October 2013, Missouri changed its protocols to allow for a compounded pentobarbital to be used in a lethal dose for executions. On November 20, 2013, Joseph Paul Franklin was executed by the state of Missouri. He was the first inmate executed in three years in the state and the first to die by a single dose of pentobarbital.

Metabolism

Pentobarbital undergoes first-pass metabolism in the liver and possibly the intestines.

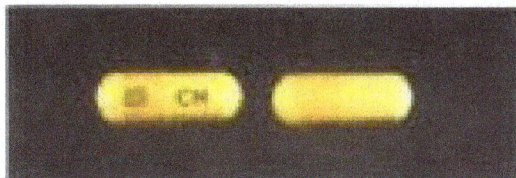

Trade Name: Nembutal
Controlled Ingredient: pentobarbital 100 mg

Drug Interactions

Administration of ethanol, benzodiazepines, opioids, antihistamines, other sedative-hypnotics, and other central nervous system depressants will cause possible additive effects.

Chemistry

Pentobarbital is synthesized by methods analogous to that of amobarbital, the only difference being that the alkylation of α-ethylmalonic ester is carried out with 2-bromopentane (not 1-bromo-3-methylbutane) to give pentobarbital.

Xylazine

Xylazine is an analogue of clonidine and an agonist at the α_2 class of adrenergic receptor. It is used for sedation, anesthesia, muscle relaxation, and analgesia in animals such as horses, cattle and other non-human mammals. Veterinarians also use xylazine as an emetic, especially in cats.

In veterinary anesthesia, xylazine is often used in combination with ketamine. It is sold under many brand names worldwide, most notably the Bayer brand name Rompun. It is also marketed as Anased, Sedazine, and Chanazine. The drug interactions vary with different animals.

It has become a drug of abuse, particularly in Puerto Rico, where it is diverted from stocks used by equine veterinarians and used as a cutting agent for heroin.

History

Xylazine was discovered as an antihypertensive agent in 1962 by Farbenfabriken Bayer in Leverkusen, Germany. Results from early human clinical studies confirmed that xylazine has several central nervous system depressant effects. Xylazine administration is used for sedation, anesthesia, muscle relaxation, and analgesia. It causes a significant reduction in blood pressure and heart rate in healthy volunteers. Due to hazardous side effects, including hypotension and bradycardia, xylazine was not approved by the Food and Drug Administration (FDA) for human use. As a result, xylazine's mechanism of action in humans remains unknown.

Xylazine was approved by the FDA for veterinary use and is now used as an animal tranquilizer. In the United States, xylazine was only approved by the FDA for veterinary use as a sedative, analgesic, and muscle relaxant in dogs, cats, horses, elk, fallow deer, mule deer, sika deer, and white-tailed deer. The sedative and analgesic effects of xylazine are related to central nervous system depression. Xylazine's muscle relaxant effect inhibits the transmission of neural impulses in the central nervous system.

In scientific research, xylazine is a component of the most common anesthetic, ketamine-xylazine, which is used in rats, mice, hamster, and guinea pigs. The accounts of the actions and uses of xylazine in animals were reported as early as the late 1960s and early 1970s. Since the early 2000s, xylazine has become popular as a drug of abuse in the United States and Puerto Rico. Xylazine's street name in Puerto Rico is *Anestesia de Caballo*, which roughly translates to "horse anesthetic." The reasons that may explain why this drug has become increasingly popular are still unknown. Further research is needed to gain more information on the distribution of xylazine in the body, physical symptoms, potential treatments, and predictive factors for chronic usage.

Medical Uses

Xylazine is often used as a sedative, muscle relaxant, and analgesic. It is frequently used in the treatment of tetanus. Xylazine is very similar to drugs such as phenothiazine, tricyclic antidepressants, and clonidine. As an anesthetic, it is typically used in conjunction with ketamine. Xylazine appears to reduce sensitivity to insulin and glucose uptake in humans. Yohimbine has been used to decrease glucose levels to a healthy level. In clinical settings, Yohimbine can reverse the adverse effects of xylazine if administered intravenously at a dosage of 0.5 mL / 20 pounds shortly after xylazine administration.

Pharmacodynamics

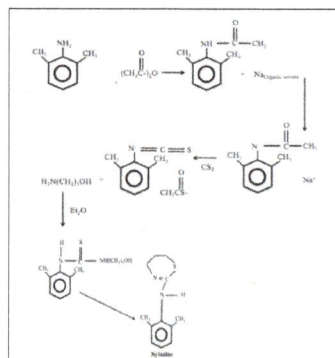

Xylazine Synthesis adapted from Elliot et al., 1986.

Xylazine is a potent α2 adrenergic agonist. When xylazine and other α2 adrenergic receptor agonists are administered, they distribute throughout the body within 30 to 40 minutes. Due to xylazine's highly lipophilic nature, xylazine directly stimulates central α2 receptors as well as peripheral α-adrenoceptors in a variety of tissues. As an agonist, xylazine leads to a decrease in neurotransmission of norepinephrine and dopamine in the central nervous system. It does so by mimicking norepinephrine in binding to presynaptic surface autoreceptors, which leads to feedback inhibition of norepinephrine.

Research has found that xylazine significantly increases Km and does not affect Vmax. Xylazine also serves as a transport inhibitor by suppressing norepinephrine transport function through competitive inhibition of substrate transport. This likely occurs by direct interaction on an area that overlaps with the antidepressant binding site. For example, xylazine and clonidine suppress uptake of MIBG, a norepinephrine analog, in neuroblastoma cells. Xylazine has varying affinities for cholinergic, serotonergic, dopaminergic, α1 adrenergic, H2 - histaminergic and opiate receptors. Its chemical structure closely resembles the phenothiazines, tricyclic antidepressants, and clonidine.

Pharmacokinetics

Xylazine is absorbed, metabolized, and eliminated rapidly. Xylazine can be inhaled or administered intravenously, intramuscularly, subcutaneously, or orally either by itself or in conjunction with other anesthetics, such as ketamine, barbiturates, chloral hydrate, and halothane in order to provide reliable anesthesia effects. The most common route of administration is injection. The drug is used as a veterinary anesthetic and the recommended dose varies between species.

If it is administered intramuscularly, the recommended dose is 0.25 – 4 mg per pound in animals. If xylazine is administered intravenously, the recommended dose is 0.5 mg per pound in animals. As a veterinary anesthetic, xylazine is typically only administered once for intended effect before or during surgical procedures. When used as a drug of abuse in humans, the frequency of dosage is dependent on social or economic factors as well as each user's subjective response to xylazine's addictive properties.

Xylazine's action can be seen usually 15 to 30 minutes after administration and the sedative effect may continue for 1–2 hours and last up to 4 hours. Once xylazine gains access to the vascular system, it is distributed within the blood, allowing xylazine to perfuse target organs including the heart, lungs, liver, and kidney. In nonfatal cases, the blood plasma concentrations range from 0.03 to 4.6 mg/L. Xylazine diffuses extensively and penetrates the blood brain barrier, as expected due to the uncharged, lipophilic nature of the compound.

In dogs, sheep, horses and cattle, the half life is very short at only 1.21 to 5.97 minutes. Complete elimination of the half lives can take up to 23.11 minutes in sheep and up to 49.51 minutes in horses. In young rats, the half life is an hour. Xylazine has a large volume of distribution (Vd). The Vd is 1.9-2.5 for horse, cattle, sheep, and dog. Though the peak plasma concentrations are reached in 12–14 minutes in all species, the bioavailability varies between species. The half life depends on the age of the animal, as age is related to prolonged duration of anesthesia and recovery time. Toxicity occurs with repeated administration, given that the metabolic clearance of the drug is usually calculated as 7 to 9 times the half-life, which is 4 to 5 days for the clearance of xylazine.

Xylazine is metabolized by liver cytochrome P450 enzymes. When it reaches the liver, xylazine is metabolized and proceeds to the kidneys to be excreted as urine. Around 70% of a dose is excreted by urine. Thus, urine can be used in detecting xylazine administration because it contains many metabolites, which are the main targets and products in urine. Within a few hours, xylazine decreases to undetectable levels. Other factors can also significantly impact the pharmacokinetics of xylazine, including sex, nutrition, environmental conditions, and prior diseases.

Xylazine Phase I Metabolites		
Xylazine-M (2,6 dimethylaniline)	Xylazine-M (N-thiourea-2,6-dimethylaniline)	Xylazine-M (sulfone-HO-) isomer 2
Xylazine-M (HO-2,6-dimethylaniline isomer 1)	Xylazine-M (HO-2,6-dimethylaniline isomer 2)	Xylazine M (oxo-)
Xylazine-M (HO-) isomer 1	Xylazine-M (HO-) isomer 1 glucuronide	Xylazine-M (HO-) isomer 2
Xylazine-M (HO-) isomer 2 glucuronide	Xylazine-M (HO-oxo-) isomer 1	Xylazine-M (HO-oxo-) isomer 1 glucuronide
Xylazine-M (HO-oxo-) isomer 2	Xylazine-M (HO-oxo-) isomer 2 glucuronide	Xylazine-M (sulfone)
	Xylazine-M (sulfone-HO-) isomer 1	

Side Effects

Humans

Xylazine overdose is usually fatal in humans. Because it is used as a drug adulterant, the symptoms caused by the drugs accompanying xylazine administration vary between individuals.

The most common side effects in humans associated with xylazine administration include bradycardia, respiratory depression, hypotension, transient hypertension secondary to vagus nerve stimulation, and other changes in cardiac output. Xylazine significantly decreases heart rate in animals that are not premedicated with medications that have anticholinergic effects. The decrease in heart rate directly impacts aortic flow. Bradycardia caused by xylazine administration is effectively prevented by administration of atropine or glycopyrrolate. Arrhythmias associated with xylazine includes other symptoms such as sinoatrial block, atrioventricular block, A-V dissociation, and sinus arrhythmia.

Xylazine administration can lead to diabetes mellitus and hyperglycemia. Other possible side effects that can occur are areflexia, asthenia, ataxia, blurred vision, disorientation, dizziness, drowsiness, dysarthria, dysmetria, fainting, hyporeflexia, slurred speech, somnolence, staggering, coma, apnea, shallow breathing, sleepiness, premature ventricular contraction, tachycardia, miosis, and dry mouth. Rarely, hypotonia, dry mouth, urinary incontinence and nonspecific electrocardiographic ST segment changes occur. It has been reported that the duration of symptoms after human overdose is 8 to 72 hours. Further research is necessary to categorize the side effects that occur when xylazine is used in conjunction with heroin and cocaine.

Chronic use is reported to be associated with physical deterioration, dependence, abscesses, and skin ulceration, which can be physically debilitating and painful. Hypertension followed by hypotension, bradycardia, and respiratory depression lower tissue oxygenation in the skin. Thus, chronic use of xylazine can progress the skin oxygenation deficit, leading to severe skin ulceration. Lower skin oxygenation is associated with impaired healing of wounds and a higher chance of infection. The ulcers may have a characteristic odor and ooze pus. In severe cases, amputations must be performed on the affected extremities.

Animals

Side effects in animals include transient hypertension, hypotension, and respiratory depression. Further, the decrease of tissue sensitivity to insulin leads to xylazine-induced hyperglycemia and a reduction of tissue glucose uptake and utilization. The duration of effects in animals lasts up to 4 hours.

Recreational Use

Xylazine users are more likely to be male, under the age of 30, living in a rural area, and injecting versus inhaling xylazine. Xylazine has similar behavioral consequences as heroin, thus it is commonly used as an adulterant. Xylazine is also frequently found in speedball. The combination of heroin and xylazine produces a stronger high than administration of heroin alone. Concomitant use of xylazine with speedball may potentiate or prolong the effects of these drugs, which can lead to adverse consequences.

Carruthers et al. in 1979 reported the first case of xylazine toxicity in a 34-year-old male, who self-medicated for insomnia with injection of 1 g of xylazine. Intentional intoxication from ingesting, inhaling, or injecting xylazine has been reported. The intravenous route is the most common route of administration for those who abuse heroin or xylazine recreationally. In Puerto Rico, xylazine has increased in popularity. Its use was associated with a high number of inmate deaths at the Guerrero Correctional Institution in Aguadilla, Puerto Rico from 2002 through 2008.

Treatment of Overdose

The known doses of xylazine that produce toxicity and fatality in humans vary from 40 to 2400 mg. Small doses may produce toxicity and larger doses may be survived with medical assistance. Non-fatal blood or plasma concentration ranges from 0.03 to 4.6 mg/L. In fatalities, the blood concentration of xylazine ranges from trace to 16 mg/L. It is reported that there is no defined safe or fatal concentration of xylazine because of the significant overlap between the non-fatal and postmortem blood concentrations of xylazine.

Currently, there is no specific antidote to treat humans that overdose on xylazine. Hemodialysis has been suggested as a form of treatment, but is usually unfavorable due to the large volume of distribution of xylazine. In addition, due to lack of research in humans, there are no standardized screenings to determine if an overdose has occurred. The detection of xylazine in biological fluids in humans involves various screening methods, such as urine screenings, thin layer chromatography (TLC), gas chromatography mass spectrometry (GC-MS), Remedi HS Bio-Rad Laboratories, and liquid chromatography mass spectrometry (LC-MS).

Multiple drugs have been used as supportive therapeutic intervention such as lidocaine, naloxone, thiamine, lorazepam, vecuronium, etomidate, propofol, tolazoline, yohimbine, atropine, naloxone, orciprenaline, metoclopramide, ranitidine, metoprolol, enoxaparin, flucloxacillin, insulin, and irrigation of both eyes with saline. Effects of xylazine are also reversed by the analeptics 4-aminopyridine, doxapram, and caffeine, which are physiological antagonists to central nervous system depressants. Combining yohimbine and 4-aminopyridine in an effort to antagonize xylazine is superior as compared to the administration of either of these drugs individually due to reduction of recovery time. Research initiatives may be necessary in order to standardize treatment and determine effective measures for identifying chronic xylazine usage and intoxication.

The treatment after xylazine overdose should primarily involve maintaining respiratory function and blood pressure. In cases of intoxication, physicians recommend intravenous fluid infusion, atropine, and hospital observation. Severe cases may require endotracheal intubation, mechanical ventilation, gastric lavage, activated charcoal, bladder catheterization, electrocardiographic (ECG) and hyperglycemia monitoring. Physicians typically recommend which detoxification treatment should be used to manage possible dysfunction involving highly perfused organs, such as the liver and kidney.

Streptomycin

Streptomycin is an antibiotic (antimycobacterial) drug, the first of a class of drugs called aminoglycosides to be discovered, and it was the first effective treatment for tuberculosis. It is derived from the actinobacterium *Streptomyces griseus*. Streptomycin is a bactericidal antibiotic. Adverse effects of this medicine are ototoxicity, nephrotoxicity, fetal auditory toxicity, and neuromuscular paralysis.

It is on the World Health Organization's List of Essential Medicines, the most important medications needed in a basic health system.

Uses

Treatment of Diseases

- Infective endocarditis caused by enterococcus when the organism is not sensitive to gentamicin

- Tuberculosis in combination with other anti-TB drugs. It is not the first-line treatment, except in medically under-served populations where the cost of more expensive treatments is prohibitive.

- Plague (*Yersinia pestis*) has historically been treated with it as the first-line treatment. However streptomycin is approved for this purpose only by the U.S. Food and Drug Administration.

- In veterinary medicine, streptomycin is the first-line antibiotic for use against gram negative bacteria in large animals (horses, cattle, sheep, etc.). It is commonly combined with procaine penicillin for intramuscular injection.

- Tularemia infections have been treated mostly with streptomycin.

Streptomycin is traditionally given intramuscularly, and in many nations is only licensed to be administered intramuscularly, though in some regions the drug may also be administered intravenously.

Pesticide and Fungicide

Streptomycin also is used as a pesticide, to combat the growth of bacteria, fungi, and algae. Streptomycin controls bacterial and fungal diseases of certain fruit, vegetables, seed, and ornamental crops, and it controls algae in ornamental ponds and aquaria. A major use is in the control of fireblight on apple and pear trees. As in medical applications, extensive use can be associated with the development of resistant strains.

Cell Culture

Streptomycin, in combination with penicillin, is used in a standard antibiotic cocktail to prevent bacterial infection in cell culture.

Protein Purification

When purifying protein from a biological extract, streptomycin sulfate is sometimes added as a means of removing nucleic acids. Since it binds to ribosomes and precipitates out of solution, it serves as a method for removing rRNA, mRNA, and even DNA if the extract is from a prokaryote.

Spectrum of Activity

Streptomycin can be used clinically to treat tuberculosis in combination with other medications and susceptible strains which cause bacterial endocarditis. The following represents MIC susceptibility for a few medically significant microorganisms.

- *Mycobacterium tuberculosis*: 1 μg/ml - 2 μg/ml

- *Staphylococcus aureus*: 4 μg/ml

Side Effects

Fever and rashes result from persistent use. The vestibular portion of cranial nerve VIII (the vestibulococlear nerve) can be affected, resulting in tinnitus, vertigo and ataxia. It can also lead to nephrotoxicity and can potentially interfere with diagnosis of kidney malfunction.

Streptomycin belongs to a class of antibiotics known as aminoglycosides which are ototoxic in some people. Aminoglycosides have been known to cause both transient and permanent hearing loss in some cases.

Mechanism of Action

Streptomycin is a protein synthesis inhibitor. It binds to the small 16S rRNA of the 30S subunit of the bacterial ribosome, interfering with the binding of formyl-methionyl-tRNA to the 30S subunit. This leads to codon misreading, eventual inhibition of protein synthesis and ultimately death of microbial cells through mechanisms that are still not understood. Speculation on this mechanism indicates that the binding of the molecule to the 30S subunit interferes with 50S subunit association with the mRNA strand. This results in an unstable ribosomal-mRNA complex, leading to a frameshift mutation and defective protein synthesis; leading to cell death. Humans have ribosomes which are structurally different from those in bacteria, so the drug does not have this effect in human cells. At low concentrations, however, streptomycin only inhibits growth of the bacteria by inducing prokaryotic ribosomes to misread mRNA. Streptomycin is an antibiotic that inhibits both Gram-positive and Gram-negative bacteria, and is therefore a useful broad-spectrum antibiotic.

History

Streptomycin was first isolated on October 19, 1943, by Albert Schatz, a graduate student, in the laboratory of Selman Abraham Waksman at Rutgers University in a research project funded by Merck and Co. Waksman and his laboratory staff discovered several antibiotics, including actinomycin, clavacin, streptothricin, streptomycin, grisein, neomycin, fradicin, candicidin, and candidin. Of these, streptomycin and neomycin found extensive application in the treatment of numerous infectious diseases. Streptomycin was the first antibiotic cure for tuberculosis (TB). In 1952 Waksman was the recipient of the Nobel Prize in Physiology or Medicine in recognition "for his discovery of streptomycin, the first antibiotic active against tuberculosis". Waksman was later accused of playing down the role of Schatz who did the work under his supervision.

At the end of World War II, the United States Army experimented with streptomycin to treat life-threatening infections at a military hospital in Battle Creek, Michigan. The first patient treated did not survive; the second patient survived but became blind as a side effect of the treatment. In March 1946, the third patient—Robert J. Dole, later Majority Leader of the United States Senate and Presidential nominee—experienced a rapid and robust recovery.

The first randomized trial of streptomycin against pulmonary tuberculosis was carried out in 1946 through 1948 by the MRC Tuberculosis Research Unit under the chairmanship of Geoffrey Marshall (1887–1982). The trial was both double-blind and placebo-controlled. It is widely accepted to have been the first randomised curative trial.

Results showed efficacy against TB, albeit with minor toxicity and acquired bacterial resistance to the drug.

Bicalutamide

Bicalutamide, sold under the brand name Casodex among others, is an antiandrogen that is used primarily in the treatment of prostate cancer. It is used alone or together with surgical or medical castration for this indication, and is able to significantly slow the course of the disease and extend life. Bicalutamide is also used to treat hirsutism (excessive hair growth in women), early-onset puberty in boys, as a component of hormone therapy for transgender women, and in the treatment of other androgen-dependent conditions.

Bicalutamide is a non-steroidal antiandrogen (NSAA) and acts as a selective antagonist of the androgen receptor (AR), the biological target of androgens like testosterone and dihydrotestosterone (DHT). It does not lower androgen levels, instead acting purely by preventing androgens from mediating their effects in the body. Bicalutamide is taken orally. It is well-absorbed, and its absorption is not affected by food. The drug has a long terminal half-life of 6 to 10 days. It crosses the blood-brain-barrier. The major side effects of bicalutamide in men are gynecomastia (breast development), breast tenderness, and feminization in general, whereas the drug produces few side effects and is very well-tolerated in women. Bicalutamide can cause elevated liver enzymes in around 1% of patients, and has been associated with a few cases of liver damage and lung toxicity in the medical literature. Monitoring of liver enzymes is recommended during treatment with bicalutamide.

Bicalutamide was developed and marketed by AstraZeneca (formerly as Imperial Chemical Industries (ICI)), and was first approved in 1995. It is the most widely used antiandrogen in the treatment of prostate cancer, as well as the most widely used NSAA, and has been prescribed to millions of men with the disease. Prior to the introduction of the newer and improved NSAA enzalutamide in 2012, bicalutamide was considered to be the standard-of-care antiandrogen in the treatment of prostate cancer. Bicalutamide shows an improved profile of effectiveness, tolerability, and safety when compared to earlier antiandrogens like the steroidal antiandrogen (SAA) cyproterone acetate (CPA) and the NSAAs flutamide and nilutamide, and has largely replaced them in the treatment of prostate cancer.

Bicalutamide is available in most developed countries, and is marketed in at least 70 countries throughout the world. Its patent protection expired in 2009 and the drug has since been available in low-cost generic formulations. Its cost is from $15.44 USD per month for a dosage of 50 mg per day. Bicalutamide is on the WHO Model List of Essential Medicines, the most important medications needed in a basic health system.

Medical Uses

Prostate Cancer

Bicalutamide is used primarily in the treatment of early and advanced prostate cancer. It is approved at a dosage of 50 mg/day as a combination therapy with a gonadotropin-releasing hormone (GnRH) analogue or orchiectomy (that is, surgical or medical castration) in the treatment of stage D2 metastatic prostate cancer (mPC), and as a monotherapy at a dosage of 150 mg/day for the treatment of stage C or D1 locally advanced prostate cancer (LAPC). Although effective in mPC and LAPC, bicalutamide is no longer indicated for the treatment of localized prostate cancer (LPC) due to negative findings in the Early Prostate Cancer (EPC) trial.

Role of Antiandrogens in Prostate Cancer

In 1941, Charles Huggins and Clarence Hodges discovered that growth of prostate cancer in men regressed with surgical castration or high-dose estrogen treatment, which were associated with very low levels of circulating testosterone, and accelerated with the administration of exogenous testosterone, findings for which they were later awarded the Nobel Prize. It has since been elucidated that androgens like testosterone and DHT function as trophic factors for the prostate gland, stimulating cell division and proliferation and producing tissue growth and glandular enlargement, which, in the context of prostate cancer, results in stimulation of tumors and a considerable acceleration of disease progression. As a result of the work of Huggins and Hodges, androgen deprivation therapy (ADT), via a variety of modalities including surgical castration, high-dose estrogens, SAAs, GnRH analogues, NSAAs, and androgen biosynthesis inhibitors (e.g., abiraterone acetate), has become the mainstay of treatment for prostate cancer. Although ADT can shrink or stabilize prostate tumors and hence significantly slow the course of prostate cancer and prolong life, it is, unfortunately, not generally curative. While effective in slowing the progression of the disease initially, most advanced prostate cancer patients eventually become resistant to ADT and prostate cancer growth starts to accelerate again, in part due to progressive mutations in the AR that result in the transformation of drugs like bicalutamide from AR antagonists to agonists.

A few scientific observations form the basis of the reasoning behind combined androgen blockade (CAB), in which castration and an NSAA are combined. It has been found that very low levels of androgens, as in castration, are able to significantly stimulate growth of prostate cancer cells and accelerate disease progression. Although castration ceases production of androgens by the gonads and reduces circulating testosterone levels by about 95%, low levels of androgens continue to be produced by the adrenal glands, and this accounts for the residual levels of circulating testosterone. Moreover, it has been found that intraprostatic levels of DHT, which is the major androgen in the prostate gland, remain at 40 to 50% of their initial values following castration. This has been determined to be due to uptake of circulating weak adrenal androgens like dehydroepiandrosterone (DHEA) and androstenedione by the prostate and their *de novo* transformation into testosterone and then DHT. As such, a significant amount of androgen signaling continues within the prostate gland even with castration. Previously, surgical adrenalectomy or therapy with older androgen biosynthesis inhibitors like ketoconazole and aminoglutethimide were successfully employed in the treatment of castration-resistant prostate cancer. However, adrenalectomy is a relatively invasive procedure with high morbidity and ketoconazole and aminoglutethimide are relatively toxic drugs, and both treatment modalities absolutely require supplementation of corticosteroids, making them in many ways unideal. The development of CAB with NSAAs like bicalutamide and enzalutamide has since allowed for a non-invasive, convenient, and well-tolerated replacement.

Subsequent clinical research has found that monotherapy with higher dosages of NSAAs than those used in CAB is slightly but non-significantly inferior or roughly equivalent to castration in extending life in men with prostate cancer. Moreover, NSAA monotherapy is overall better tolerated and associated with greater quality of life than is castration, which is thought to be related to the fact that testosterone levels do not decrease with NSAA monotherapy and hence by extension that levels of biologically active and beneficial metabolites of testosterone such as estrogens and neurosteroids are preserved. For these reasons, NSAA monotherapy has become an important alternative to castration and CAB in the treatment of prostate cancer.

Other Uses

Excess Hair and Acne

Low-dose bicalutamide has been found to be effective in the treatment of hirsutism (excessive body and/or facial hair growth) in women in at least three clinical studies. [*unreliable medical source*] In one such study, the drug was well-tolerated, all of the patients experienced a visible decrease in hair density, and a highly significant clinical improvement was observed with the Ferriman–Gallwey score decreasing by 41.2% at 3 months and by 61.6% at 6 months. According to a recent review, "Low dose bicalutamide (25 mg/day) was shown to be effective in the treatment of hirsutism related to IH and PCOS. It does not have any significant side effects [or lead] to irregular periods."

In addition to hirsutism, bicalutamide can also be used in the treatment of acne in women. Several studies have observed complete clearing of acne with flutamide in women, and similar or benefits would be expected with bicalutamide.Bicalutamide may also treat other androgen-dependent skin conditions, such as seborrhea and androgenic alopecia (pattern hair loss). Flutamide has been found to produce a decrease of hirsutism score to normal and an 80% or greater decrease in scores of acne, seborrhea, and androgen-dependent hair loss. Moreover, in combination with an oral contraceptive, flutamide treatment resulted in an increase in cosmetically acceptable scalp hair density in 6 of 7 women suffering from androgenic alopecia.

Transgender Hormone Therapy

Bicalutamide is used as a component of hormone replacement therapy (HRT) in the endocrinological treatment of transgender women. Beneficial or desired effects include breast development, reduced male-pattern hair, decreased muscle mass, changes in fat distribution, lowered libido, and loss of spontaneous erections. Bicalutamide monotherapy increases estradiol levels in biological males and hence has indirect estrogenic effects in transgender women. This is a property that can be considered to be desirable in transgender women, as it produces or contributes to feminization.

Unlike the cases of the SAAs spironolactone and CPA and GnRH analogues, no clinical studies assessing bicalutamide as an antiandrogen in the hormonal treatment of transgender women have been published. However, bicalutamide is effective as an antiandrogen in women (with hirsutism) and in boys with precocious puberty, and feminization is a well-documented effect of bicalutamide in men treated with it for prostate cancer. In addition, nilutamide, which is a closely related antiandrogen that possesses the same mechanism of action as bicalutamide, *has* been evaluated in transgender women in at least five small clinical studies. In these studies, nilutamide monotherapy (i.e., without estrogen), employed at the same dosage at which it is used in prostate cancer (300 mg/day), induced observable signs of clinical feminization in young transgender women (age range 19–33 years) within 8 weeks, including breast development, decreased male-pattern hair, decreased morning erections and sex drive, and positive psychological and emotional changes. Signs of breast development occurred in all subjects within 6 weeks and were associated with increased nipple sensitivity, and along with decreased hair growth, were the earliest sign of feminization. The drug more than doubled luteinizing hormone (LH) and testosterone levels and tripled estradiol levels , and the addition of ethinyl estradiol (a potent estrogen) to nilutamide therapy after 8 weeks of treatment abolished the increase in LH, testosterone, and estradiol levels and dramatically suppressed testosterone levels, into the castrate range. Both nilutamide alone and particularly the combination of nilutamide and estrogen were regarded as effective in terms of antiandrogen action and producing feminization in transgender women. However, use of nilutamide itself for prostate cancer and other conditions is now discouraged due to its unique adverse effects, most importantly a high incidence of interstitial pneumonitis (which can progress to pulmonary fibrosis and potentially be fatal), and newer, safer NSAAs like bicalutamide and enzalutamide have largely replaced it and are used instead.

According to Dr. Madeline Deutsch of the Center of Excellence for Transgender Health (a division of the University of California, San Francisco) in the *Guidelines for the Primary and Gender-Affirming Care of Transgender and Gender Nonbinary People* (2016), on the topic of bicalutamide in transgender women:

In many countries, cyproterone acetate, a synthetic progestagen with strong anti-androgen activity is commonly used [as an antiandrogen in feminizing hormone therapy for transgender women]. Cyproterone [acetate] has been associated with uncommon episodes of fulminant hepatitis. Bicalutamide, a direct anti-androgen used for the treatment of prostate cancer, also has a small but not fully quantified risk of liver function abnormalities (including several cases of fulminant hepatitis); while such risks are acceptable when considering the benefits of bicalutamide in the management of prostate cancer, such risks are less justified in the context of gender-affirming treatment. No evidence at present exists to inform such an analysis.

It is noteworthy, however, that CPA is widely used as an antiandrogen for the treatment of transgender women (and cisgender women with acne and hirsutism) outside of the U.S. (a country where CPA is unavailable and spironolactone is generally used instead) yet appears to have a much higher comparative risk of hepatotoxicity than does bicalutamide. Only five cases of hepatotoxicity have been associated with bicalutamide to date.

Male Early Puberty

Bicalutamide (25–50 mg/day) is useful in combination with the aromatase inhibitor anastrozole as a puberty blocker in the treatment of male precocious puberty. This is potentially a cost-effective alternative to GnRH analogues for the treatment of this condition, as GnRH analogues are very expensive. Moreover, the combination is effective in gonadotropin-independent precocious puberty, namely familial male-limited precocious puberty (also known as testotoxicosis), where GnRH analogues notably are not effective. Bicalutamide has been found to be superior to the SAA spironolactone (which has also been used, in combination with the aromatase inhibitor testolactone) for this indication; it has shown greater effectiveness and possesses fewer side effects in comparison. For this reason, bicalutamide has replaced spironolactone in the treatment of the condition.

Priapism

Antiandrogens can considerably relieve and prevent priapism (potentially painful penile erections that last more than four hours) via direct blockade of penile ARs. In accordance, bicalutamide, at low dosages (50 mg every other day or as little as once or twice weekly), has been found in a series of case reports to completely resolve recurrent priapism in men without producing significant side effects, and is used for this indication off-label. In the reported cases, libido, rigid erections, the potential for sexual intercourse, orgasm, and subjective ejaculatory volume have all remained intact or unchanged, and gynecomastia has not developed when bicalutamide is administered at a total dosage of 25 mg/day or less. Some gynecomastia and breast tenderness developed in one patient treated with 50 mg/day, but significantly improved upon the dosage being halved. The observed tolerability profile of bicalutamide in these subjects has been regarded as significantly more favorable than that of GnRH analogues and estrogens (which are also used in the treatment of this condition). However, although successful and well-tolerated, very few cases have been reported.

Available Forms

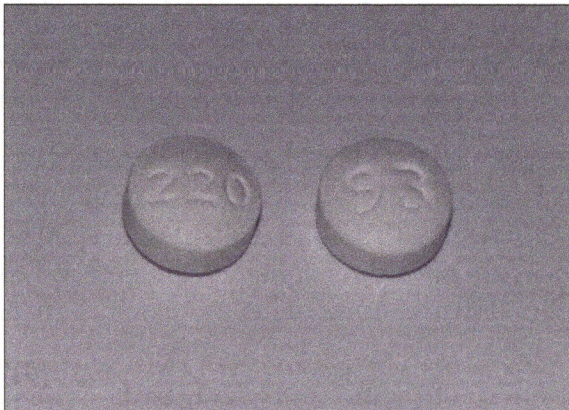

Bicalutamide Teva 50 mg tablets.

Bicalutamide is available in 50 mg, 80 mg (in Japan), and 150 mg tablets for oral administration. No other formulations or routes of administration are available or used. All formulations of bicalutamide are specifically indicated for the treatment of prostate cancer alone or in combination with surgical or medication castration.

A combined formulation of bicalutamide and the GnRH agonist goserelin in which goserelin is provided as a subcutaneous implant for injection and bicalutamide is included as 50 mg tablets for oral ingestion is marketed in Australia and New Zealand under the brand name ZolaCos CP (*Zoladex-Cosudex Combination Pack*).

Contraindications

Hepatic Impairment

In individuals with severe, though not mild-to-moderate hepatic impairment, there is evidence that the elimination of bicalutamide is slowed, and hence, caution may be warranted in these patients. In severe hepatic impairment, the terminal half-life of the active (R)-enantiomer of bicalutamide is increased by about 1.75-fold (76% increase; half-life of 5.9 and 10.4 days for normal and impaired patients, respectively). The terminal half-life of bicalutamide is unchanged in renal impairment.

Pregnancy and Breastfeeding

Because bicalutamide blocks the AR, like all antiandrogens, it can interfere with the androgen-mediated sexual differentiation of the genitalia (and brain) during prenatal development. In pregnant rats given bicalutamide at a dosage of 10 mg/kg/day (resulting in circulating drug levels approximately equivalent to two-thirds of human therapeutic concentrations) and above, feminization of male offspring, such as reduced anogenital distance and hypospadias, as well as impotence, were observed. No other teratogenic effects were observed in rats or rabbits receiving up to very high dosages of bicalutamide (that corresponded to up to approximately two times human therapeutic levels), and no teratogenic effects of any sort were observed in female rat offspring at any dosage. As such, bicalutamide is a reproductive teratogen in males, and may have the potential to produce undervirilization/sexually ambiguous genitalia in male fetuses. For this reason, the drug is contraindicated in women during pregnancy, and women who are sexually active and who can or may become pregnant are strongly recommended to take bicalutamide only in combination with contraception. It is unknown whether bicalutamide is excreted in breast milk, but many drugs are excreted in breast milk, and for this reason, breastfeeding is not recommended during bicalutamide treatment.

Side Effects

The side effect profile of bicalutamide is highly sex-dependent. In women, the side effects of pure antiandrogens/NSAAs are minimal, and bicalutamide has been found to be very well-tolerated. In men however, due to androgen deprivation, a variety of side effects of varying severity may occur during bicalutamide treatment, with breast pain/tenderness and gynecomastia being the most common and others including physical feminization and demasculinization in general (e.g., reduced body hair growth/density, decreased muscle mass and strength, changes in fat mass and distribution, and reduced penile length), hot flashes, sexual dysfunction (including loss of libido and erectile dysfunction), depression, fatigue, weakness, anemia, and decreased semen/ejaculate volume. General side effects of bicalutamide that may occur in either sex may include diarrhea, constipation, abdominal pain, nausea, dry skin, itching, and rash. The drug is well-tolerated at higher dosages (than the 50 mg/day dosage), with rare additional side effects.

Gynecomastia

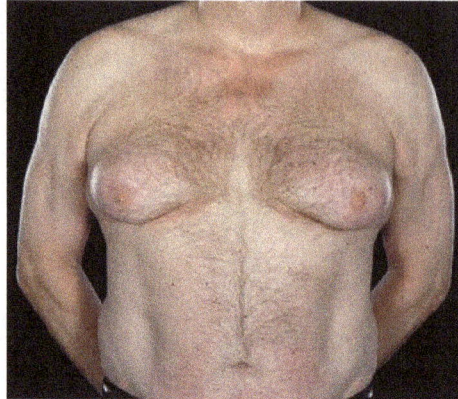

Gynecomastia in a 60-year-old man treated with 150 mg/day bicalutamide for prostate cancer.

The most common side effects of bicalutamide monotherapy in men are breast pain/tenderness and gynecomastia. These side effects may occur in up to more than 90% of men treated with bicalutamide monotherapy, but gynecomastia is generally reported to occur in 70–80% of patients. In the EPC trial, at a median follow-up of 7.4 years, breast pain and gynecomastia respectively occurred in 73.6% and 68.8% of men treated with 150 mg/day bicalutamide monotherapy. In more than 90% of affected men, bicalutamide-related breast events are mild-to-moderate in severity. It is only rarely and in severe or extreme cases of gynecomastia that the proportions of the male breasts become so marked that they are comparable to those of women. In the EPC trial, 16.8% of bicalutamide patients relative to 0.7% of controls withdrew from the study due to breast pain and/or gynecomastia. The incidence and severity of gynecomastia are higher with estrogens (e.g., diethylstilbestrol) than with NSAAs like bicalutamide in the treatment of men with prostate cancer.

Management

Tamoxifen, a selective estrogen receptor modulator (SERM) with antiestrogenic actions in breast tissue and estrogenic actions in bone, has been found to be highly effective in preventing and reversing bicalutamide-induced gynecomastia in men. Moreover, in contrast to GnRH analogues (which also alleviate bicalutamide-induced gynecomastia), tamoxifen poses minimal risk of accelerated bone loss and osteoporosis. For reasons that are unclear, anastrozole, an aromatase inhibitor (or an inhibitor of estrogen biosynthesis), has been found to be much less effective in comparison to tamoxifen for treating bicalutamide-induced gynecomastia. A systematic review of NSAA-induced gynecomastia and breast tenderness concluded that tamoxifen (10–20 mg/day) and radiotherapy could effectively manage the side effect without relevant adverse effects, though with tamoxifen showing superior effectiveness. Surgical breast reduction may also be employed to correct bicalutamide-induced gynecomastia.

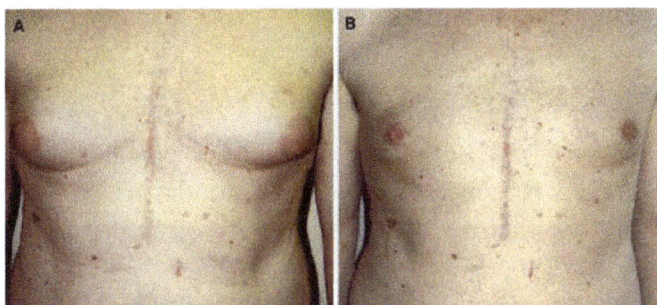

Severe gynecomastia in a 64-year-old man treated with 150 mg/day bicalutamide for prostate cancer. Before (A) and after (B) surgical breast reduction.

Sexual Dysfunction

Bicalutamide may cause sexual dysfunction, including decreased sex drive and erectile dysfunction. However, the rates of these side effects with bicalutamide monotherapy are very low. In the EPC trial, at 7.4 years follow-up, the rates of decreased libido and impotence were only 3.6% and 9.3% in the 150 mg/day bicalutamide monotherapy group relative to 1.2% and 6.5% for placebo, respectively. Most men experience sexual dysfunction only moderately or not at all with bicalutamide monotherapy, and the same is true during monotherapy with other NSAAs. In clinical trials, about two-thirds of men with advanced prostate cancer (and of almost invariably advanced age) treated with bicalutamide monotherapy maintained sexual interest, while sexual function was slightly reduced by 18%.

Reproductive Changes

Bicalutamide reduces the size of the prostate gland and seminal vesicles, though not of the testes. Significantly reduced penile length is also a recognized adverse effect of ADT. Reversible hypospermia or aspermia (that is, reduced or absent semen/ejaculate production) may occur. However, bicalutamide does not appear to adversely affect spermatogenesis, and thus may not necessarily abolish the capacity/potential for fertility in men. Due to the induction of chronic overproduction of LH and testosterone, there was concern that long-term bicalutamide monotherapy might induce Leydig cell hyperplasia and tumors (usually benign), but the evidence indicates that Leydig cell hyperplasia does not occur to a significant extent.

Other Side Effects

Gastrointestinal

The incidence of diarrhea with bicalutamide monotherapy in the EPC trial was comparable to placebo (6.3% vs. 6.4%, respectively). In phase III studies of bicalutamide monotherapy for LAPC, the rates of diarrhea for bicalutamide and castration were 6.4% and 12.5%, respectively, the rates of constipation were 13.7% and 14.4%, respectively, and the rates of abdominal pain were 10.5% and 5.6%, respectively.

Hot Flashes

In the EPC trial, at 7.4 years follow-up, the rate of hot flashes was 9.2% for bicalutamide relative to 5.4% for placebo, which was regarded as relatively low. In the LAPC subgroup of the EPC trial, the rate of hot flashes with bicalutamide was 13.1% (relative to 50.0% for castration).

Depression and Asthenia

At 5.3 years follow-up, the incidence of depression was 5.5% for bicalutamide relative to 3.0% for placebo in the EPC trial, and the incidence of asthenia (weakness or fatigue) was 10.2% for bicalutamide relative to 5.1% for placebo.

Anemia

Androgens are known to stimulate the formation of red blood cells, and for this reason, whether via castration, NSAA monotherapy, or CAB, mild anemia is a common side effect of ADT in men. The incidence of anemia with bicalutamide as a monotherapy or with castration was about 7.4% in clinical trials. A decrease of hemoglobin levels of 1–2 g/dL after approximately six months of treatment may be observed.

Skin Changes

Androgens are involved in regulation of the skin (e.g., sebum production), and antiandrogens are known to be associated with skin changes. Skin-related side effects, which included dry skin, itching, and rash, were reported at a rate of 12% in both monotherapy and CAB clinical studies of bicalutamide in men.

With Castration

Combination of bicalutamide with medical (i.e., a GnRH analogue) or surgical castration modifies the side effect profile of bicalutamide. Some of its side effects, including breast pain/tenderness and gynecomastia, are far less likely to occur when the drug is combined with a GnRH analogue, while certain other side effects, including hot flashes, depression, fatigue, and sexual dysfunction, occur much more frequently in combination with a GnRH analogue. It is thought that this is due to the suppression of estrogen levels (in addition to androgen levels) by GnRH analogues, as estrogen may compensate for various negative central effects of androgen deprivation. If bicalutamide is combined with a GnRH analogue or surgical castration, the elevation of androgen and estrogen levels in men caused by bicalutamide will be prevented and the side effects of excessive estrogens, namely gynecomastia, will be reduced. However, due to the loss of estrogen, bone loss will accelerate and the risk of osteoporosis developing with long-term therapy will increase.

Increased Mortality

In the LPC group of the EPC study, although 150 mg/day bicalutamide monotherapy had reduced mortality due to prostate cancer relative to placebo, there was a trend toward significantly increased overall mortality for bicalutamide relative to placebo at 5.4-year follow-up (25.2% vs. 20.5%). This was because more bicalutamide than placebo recipients had died due to causes unrelated to prostate cancer in this group (16.8% vs. 9.5% at 5.4-year follow-up; 10.2% vs. 9.2% at 7.4-year follow-up). At 7.4-year follow-up, there were numerically more deaths from heart failure (1.2% vs. 0.6%; 49 vs. 25 patients) and gastrointestinal cancer (1.3% vs. 0.9%) in the bicalutamide group relative to placebo recipients, although cardiovascular morbidity was similar between the two groups and there was no consistent pattern suggestive of drug-related toxicity for bicalutamide. In any case, although the reason for the increased overall mortality with 150 mg/day bicalutamide monotherapy has not been fully elucidated, it has been said that the finding that heart failure was twice as frequent in the bicalutamide group warrants further investigation. In this regard, it is notable that low testosterone levels in men have been associated in epidemiological studies with cardiovascular disease as well as with a variety of other disease states (including hypertension, hypercholesterolemia, diabetes, obesity, Alzheimer's disease, osteoporosis, and frailty).

According to Iversen et al. (2006), the increased non-prostate cancer mortality with bicalutamide monotherapy in LPC patients has also been seen with castration (via orchiectomy or GnRH analogue monotherapy) and is likely a consequence of androgen deprivation in men rather than a specific drug toxicity of bicalutamide:

The increased number of deaths in patients with localized disease receiving bicalutamide was meticulously investigated and they appeared to be due to a number of small imbalances rather than a specific cause. In addition, no direct toxic effect on any organ system could be identified. From this it may be speculated that the excess deaths in patients who are at low risk from prostate cancer mortality reflect the impact of endocrine therapy (rather than bicalutamide in particular). [...] The increased number of non-prostate cancer deaths in the early castration therapy arm [(via orchiectomy or GnRH monotherapy)] in the [Medical Research Council] study suggests that the trend towards an increased number of deaths in patients with localized disease in the present study is a reflection of early endocrine therapy as a concept rather than a bicalutamide-related phenomenon.

Rare Reactions

Livertcity

Bicalutamide may cause liver changes rarely, such as elevated transaminases (a marker of hepatotoxicity) and jaundice. In the EPC study of 4,052 prostate cancer patients who received 150 mg/day bicalutamide as a monotherapy, the incidence of abnormal liver function tests was 3.4% for bicalutamide and 1.9% for standard care (a 1.5% difference potentially attributable to bicalutamide) at 3-year median follow-up. For comparison, the incidences of abnormal liver function tests are 42–62% for flutamide, 2–3% for nilutamide, and (dose-dependently) between 9.6% and 28.2% for CPA, whereas there appears to be no risk with enzalutamide. In the EPC trial, bicalutamide-induced liver changes were usually transient and rarely severe. The drug was discontinued due to liver changes (manifested as hepatitis or marked increases in liver enzymes) in approximately 0.3% to 1% of patients treated with it for prostate cancer in clinical trials.

The risk of liver changes with bicalutamide is considered to be small but significant, and monitoring of liver function is recommended. Elevation of transaminases above twice the normal range or jaundice may be an indication that bicalutamide should be discontinued. Liver changes with bicalutamide usually occur within the first 3 or 4 months of treatment, and it is recommended that liver function be monitored regularly for the first 4 months of treatment and periodically thereafter. Symptoms that may indicate liver dysfunction include nausea, vomiting, abdominal pain, fatigue, anorexia, "flu-like" symptoms, dark urine, and jaundice.

Out of millions of patient exposures, a total of five cases of bicalutamide-associated hepatotoxicity or liver failure, two of which were fatal, have been reported in the medical literature as of 2016. One of these cases occurred after only two doses of bicalutamide, and has been regarded as much more likely to have been caused by prolonged prior exposure of the patient to flutamide and CPA. In the five reported cases of bicalutamide-associated hepatotoxicity, the dosages of the drug were 50 mg/day (three), 100 mg/day (one), and 150 mg/day (one). Relative to flutamide (which has an estimated incidence rate of 3 in every 10,000), hepatotoxicity or liver failure is far rarer with bicalutamide and nilutamide, and bicalutamide is regarded as having the lowest risk of the three drugs. For comparison, by 1996, 46 cases of severe cholestatic hepatitis associated with flutamide had been reported, with 20 of the cases resulting in death. Moreover, a 2002 review reported that there were 18 reports of hepatotoxicity associated with CPA in the medical literature, with 6 of the reported cases resulting in death, and the review also cited a report of an additional 96 instances of hepatotoxicity that were attributed to CPA, 33 of which resulted in death.

From a theoretical standpoint (on the basis of structure-activity relationships), it has been suggested that flutamide, bicalutamide, and nilutamide, to varying extents, all have the potential to cause liver toxicity. However, in contrast to flutamide, hydroxyflutamide, and nilutamide, bicalutamide exhibits much less or no mitochondrial toxicity and inhibition of enzymes in the electron transport chain such as respiratory complex I (NADH ubiquinone oxidoreductase), and this may be the reason for its much lower risk of hepatotoxicity in comparison. The activity difference may be related to the fact that flutamide, hydroxyflutamide, and nilutamide all possess a nitroaromatic group, whereas in bicalutamide, a cyano group is present in place of this nitro group, potentially reducing toxicity.

Lung Toxicity

Several case reports of interstitial pneumonitis (which can progress to pulmonary fibrosis) in association with bicalutamide treatment have been published in the medical literature. Interstitial pneumonitis with bicalutamide is said to be an extremely rare event, and the risk is far less relative to that seen with nilutamide (which has an incidence rate of 0.5–2% of patients). In a very large cohort of prostate cancer patients, the incidence of interstitial pneumonitis with NSAAs was 0.77% for nilutamide but only 0.04% for flutamide and 0.01% for bicalutamide. An assessment done prior to the publication of the aforementioned study estimated the rates of pulmonary toxicity with flutamide, bicalutamide, and nilutamide as 1 case, 5 cases, and 303 cases per million, respectively. In addition to interstitial pneumonitis, a single case report of eosinophilic lung disease in association with six months of 200 mg/day bicalutamide treatment exists. Side effects associated with the rare potential pulmonary adverse reactions of bicalutamide may include dyspnea (difficult breathing or shortness of breath), cough, and pharyngitis (inflammation of the pharynx, resulting in sore throat).

Photosensitivity

A few cases of photosensitivity (hypersensitivity to ultraviolet light-induced skin redness and/or lesions) associated with bicalutamide have been reported. In one of the cases, bicalutamide was continued due to effectiveness in treating prostate cancer in the patient, and in combination with strict photoprotection (in the form of avoidance/prevention of ultraviolet light exposure), the symptoms disappeared and did not recur. Flutamide is also associated with photosensitivity, but much more frequently in comparison to bicalutamide.

Hypersensitivity

Hypersensitivity reactions (i.e., drug allergy), including angioedema and hives, have uncommonly been reported with bicalutamide.

Male Breast cancer

A case report of male breast cancer subsequent to bicalutamide-induced gynecomastia has been published. According to the authors, "this is the second confirmed case of breast cancer in association with bicalutamide-induced gynaecomastia (correspondence AstraZeneca)." It is notable, however, that gynecomastia does not seem to increase the risk of breast cancer in men. Moreover, the lifetime incidence of breast cancer in men is approximately 0.1%, the average age of diagnosis of prostate cancer and male breast cancer are similar (around 70 years), and millions of men have been treated with bicalutamide for prostate cancer, all of which are potentially in support of the notion of chance co-occurrences. In accordance, the authors concluded that "causality cannot be established" and that it was "probable that the association is entirely coincidental and sporadic."

Overdose

A single oral dose of bicalutamide in humans that results in symptoms of overdose or that is considered to be life-threatening has not been established. Dosages of up to 600 mg/day have been well-tolerated in clinical trials, and it is notable that there is a saturation of absorption with bicalutamide such that circulating levels of its active (*R*)-enantiomer do not further increase above a dosage of 300 mg/day. Overdose is considered to be unlikely to be life-threatening with bicalutamide or other first-generation NSAAs (i.e., flutamide and nilutamide). A massive overdose of nilutamide (13 grams, or 43 times the normal maximum 300 mg/day clinical dosage) in a 79-year-old man was uneventful, producing no clinical signs or symptoms or toxicity. There is no specific antidote for bicalutamide or NSAA overdose, and treatment should be based on symptoms.

Interactions

Cytochrome P450 Enzymes

Bicalutamide is almost exclusively metabolized by CYP3A4. As such, its levels in the body may be altered by inhibitors and inducers of CYP3A4. However, in spite of the fact bicalutamide is metabolized by CYP3A4, there is no evidence of clinically significant drug interactions when bicalutamide at a dosage of 150 mg/day or less is co-administered with drugs that inhibit or induce cytochrome P450 enzyme activity.

Plasma Binding Proteins

Because bicalutamide circulates at relatively high concentrations and is highly protein-bound, it has the potential to displace other highly protein-bound drugs like warfarin, phenytoin, theophylline, and aspirin from plasma binding proteins. This could, in turn, result in increased free concentrations of such drugs and increased effects and/or side effects, potentially necessitating dosage adjustments. Bicalutamide has specifically been found to displace coumarin anticoagulants like warfarin from their plasma binding proteins (namely albumin) *in vitro*, potentially resulting in an increased anticoagulant effect, and for this reason, close monitoring of prothrombin time and dosage adjustment as necessary is recommended when bicalutamide is used in combination with these drugs. However, in spite of this, no conclusive evidence of an interaction between bicalutamide and other drugs was found in clinical trials of nearly 3,000 patients.

Comparison with Other Antiandrogens

Since their introduction, bicalutamide and the other NSAAs have largely replaced CPA, an older drug and an SAA, in the treatment of prostate cancer. Bicalutamide was the third NSAA to be marketed, with flutamide and nilutamide preceding, and followed by enzalutamide. Relative to the earlier antiandrogens, bicalutamide has substantially reduced toxicity, and in contrast to them, is said to have an excellent and favorable safety profile. For these reasons, as well as superior potency, tolerability, and pharmacokinetics, bicalutamide is preferred and has largely replaced flutamide and nilutamide in clinical practice. In accordance, bicalutamide is the most widely used antiandrogen in the treatment of prostate cancer. Between January 2007 and December 2009, it accounted in the U.S. for about 87.2% of NSAA prescriptions. Prior to the 2012 approval of enzalutamide, a newer and improved NSAA with greater potency and efficacy, bicalutamide was regarded as the standard-of-care antiandrogen in the treatment of the prostate cancer.

First-generation NSAAs

Comparison of first-generation NSAAs			
Property	**Flutamide**	**Nilutamide**	**Bicalutamide**
Half-life	5–6 hours	~2 days	~7 days
AR RBA	25%	20%	100%
Dosage	250 mg t.i.d.	100 mg t.i.d.	150 mg o.d.
Unique side effects/ risks	• Diarrhea • Hepatotoxicity • Photosensitivity	• Nausea and vomiting • Visual disturbances • Alcohol intolerance • Interstitial pneumonitis	• None

Flutamide and nilutamide are first-generation NSAAs, similarly to bicalutamide, and all three drugs possess the same core mechanism of action of being selective AR antagonists. However, bicalutamide is the most potent of the three, with the highest affinity for the AR and the longest half-life, and is the safest, least toxic, and best-tolerated. For these reasons, bicalutamide has largely replaced flutamide and nilutamide in clinical use, and is by far the most widely used first-generation NSAA.

Effectiveness

In terms of binding to the AR, the active (R)-enantiomer of bicalutamide has 4-fold greater affinity relative to that of hydroxyflutamide, the active metabolite of flutamide (a prodrug), and 5-fold higher affinity relative to that of nilutamide. In addition, bicalutamide possesses the longest half-life of the three drugs, with half-lives of 6–10 days for bicalutamide, 5–6 hours for flutamide and 8–9 hours for hydroxyflutamide, and 23–87 hours (mean 56 hours) for nilutamide. Due to the relatively short half-lives of flutamide and hydroxyflutamide, flutamide must be taken three times daily at 8-hour intervals, whereas bicalutamide and nilutamide may be taken once daily. For this reason, dosing of bicalutamide (and nilutamide) is more convenient than with flutamide. The greater AR affinity and longer half-life of bicalutamide allow it to be used at relatively low dosages in comparison to flutamide (750–1500 mg/day) and nilutamide (150–300 mg/day) in the treatment of prostate cancer.

While it has not been directly compared to nilutamide, the effectiveness of bicalutamide has been found to be at least equivalent to that of flutamide in the treatment of prostate cancer in a direct head-to-head comparison. Moreover, indications of superior efficacy, including significantly greater relative decreases and increases in levels of prostate-specific antigen (PSA) and testosterone, respectively, were observed.

It has been reported that hydroxyflutamide and nilutamide, in contrast to bicalutamide, have some ability to weakly activate the AR at high concentrations.

Tolerability and Safety

Tolerability of NSAAs based on clinical data (Buzzatti et al., 2014)				
Side effect	Flutamide	Nilutamide	Bicalutamide	Enzalutamide
Fatigue	–	–	+	++
Hepatotoxicity	+	–	–	–
Diarrhea	++	–	+	+
Nausea	+	++	–	+
Constipation	–	–	+	+
Gynecomastia	+++	+++	+++	++
Breast pain	+++	+++	+++	++
Hot flashes	++	–	+	+
Seizures	–	–	–	+
Hypertension	–	–	–	+
Visual disturbances	–	++	–	–
Alcohol intolerance	–	+	–	–
Back pain	–	–	+	+
–: Not reported; +: ≥ 1%, < 20%; ++: ≥ 20%, < 40%; +++: ≥ 40%				

The core side effects of NSAAs such as gynecomastia, sexual dysfunction, and hot flashes occur at similar rates with the different drugs. Conversely, bicalutamide is associated with a significantly lower rate of diarrhea compared to flutamide. In fact, the incidence of diarrhea did not differ between the bicalutamide and placebo groups (6.3% vs. 6.4%, respectively) in the EPC trial, whereas diarrhea occurs in up to 20% of patients treated with flutamide. The rate of nausea and vomiting appears to be lower with bicalutamide and flutamide than with nilutamide (approximately 30% incidence of nausea with nilutamide, usually rated as mild-to-moderate). In addition, bicalutamide (and flutamide) is not associated with alcohol intolerance, visual disturbances, or a high rate of interstitial pneumonitis. In terms of toxicity and rare reactions, as described above, bicalutamide appears to have the lowest relative risks of hepatotoxicity and interstitial pneumonitis, with respective incidences far below those of flutamide and nilutamide. In contrast to flutamide and nilutamide, no specific complications have been linked to bicalutamide.

Cost

The patent protection of all three of the first-generation NSAAs has expired and flutamide and bicalutamide are both available as relatively inexpensive generics. Nilutamide, on the other hand, has always been a poor third competitor to flutamide and bicalutamide and, in relation to this fact, has not been developed as a generic and is only available as brand name Nilandron, at least in the U.S.

Second-generation NSAAs

Enzalutamide, along with the in-development apalutamide and darolutamide, are newer, second-generation NSAAs. Similarly to bicalutamide and the other first-generation NSAAs, they possess the same core mechanism of action of selective AR antagonism, but are considerably more potent and efficacious in comparison.

Effectiveness

In comparison to bicaclutamide, enzalutamide has 5- to 8-fold higher affinity for the AR, possesses mechanistic differences resulting in improved AR deactivation, shows increased (though by no means complete) resistance to AR mutations in prostate cancer cells causing a switch from antagonist to agonist activity, and has an even longer half-life (8–9 days versus ~6 days for bicalutamide). In accordance, enzalutamide, at a dosage of 160 mg/day, has been found to produce similar increases in testosterone, estradiol, and LH levels relative to high-dosage bicalutamide (300 mg/day), and an almost two-fold higher increase in testosterone levels relative to 150 mg/day bicalutamide (114% versus 66%). These findings suggest that enzalutamide is a significantly more potent and effective antiandrogen in comparison. Moreover, the drug has demonstrated superior clinical effectiveness in the treatment of prostate cancer in a direct head-to-head comparison with bicalutamide.

Tolerability and Safety

In terms of tolerability, enzalutamide and bicalutamide appear comparable in most regards, with a similar moderate negative effect on sexual function and activity for instance. However, enzalutamide has a risk of seizures and other central side effects such as anxiety and insomnia related to off-target $GABA_A$ receptor inhibition that bicalutamide does not appear to have. On the other hand, unlike with all of the earlier NSAAs (flutamide, nilutamide, and bicalutamide), there has been no evidence of hepatotoxicity or elevated liver enzymes in association with enzalutamide treatment in clinical trials. In addition to differences in adverse effects, enzalutamide is a strong inducer of CYP3A4 and a moderate inducer of CYP2C9 and CYP2C19 and poses a high risk of major drug interactions (CYP3A4 alone being involved in the metabolism of approximately 50 to 60% of clinically important drugs), whereas drug interactions are few and minimal with bicalutamide.

Cost

Unlike bicalutamide, enzalutamide is still on-patent, and for this reason, is extremely expensive ($7,450 USD for a 30-day supply as of 2015). In contrast, bicalutamide is off-patent and available as a generic, and its cost is very low in comparison (from $15.44 for a 30-day supply of once-daily 50 mg tablets).

Steroidal Antiandrogens

SAAs include CPA, megestrol acetate, chlormadinone acetate, and spironolactone. These drugs are steroids, and similarly to NSAAs, act as competitive antagonists of the AR, reducing androgenic activity in the body. In contrast to NSAAs however, they are non-selective, also binding to other steroid hormone receptors, and exhibit a variety of other activities including progestogenic, antigonadotropic, glucocorticoid, and/or antimineralocorticoid. In addition, they are not silent antagonists of the AR, but are rather weak partial agonists with the capacity for both antiandrogenic and androgenic actions. Of the SAAs, CPA is the only one that has been widely used in the treatment of prostate cancer. As antiandrogens, the SAAs have largely been replaced by the NSAAs and are now rarely used in the treatment of prostate cancer, due to the superior selectivity, efficacy, and tolerability profiles of NSAAs. However, some of them, namely CPA and spironolactone, are still commonly used in the management of certain androgen-dependent conditions (e.g., acne and hirsutism in women) and as the antiandrogen component of HRT for transgender women.

Effectiveness

In a large-scale clinical trial that compared 750 mg/day flutamide and 250 mg/day CPA monotherapies in the treatment of men with prostate cancer, the two drugs were found to have equivalent effectiveness on all endpoints. In addition, contrarily to the case of men, flutamide has been found in various clinical studies to be more effective than CPA (and particularly spironolactone) in the treatment of androgen-dependent conditions such as acne and hirsutism in women. This difference in effectiveness in men and women may be related to the fact that NSAAs like flutamide significantly increase androgen levels in men, which counteracts their antiandrogen potency, but do not increase androgen levels in women. (In contrast to NSAAs, CPA, due to its progestogenic and hence antigonadotropic activity, does not increase and rather suppresses androgen levels in both sexes.)

Bicalutamide has been found to be at least as effective as or more effective than flutamide in the treatment of prostate cancer, and is considered to be the most powerful antiandrogen of the three first-generation NSAAs. As such, although bicalutamide has not been compared head-to-head to CPA or spironolactone in the treatment of androgen-dependent conditions, flutamide has been found to be either equivalent or more effective than them in clinical studies, and the same would consequently be expected of bicalutamide. Accordingly, a study comparing the efficacy of 50 mg/day bicalutamide versus 300 mg/day CPA in preventing the PSA flare at the start of GnRH agonist therapy in men with prostate cancer found that the two regimens were equivalently effective. There was evidence of a slight advantage in terms of speed of onset and magnitude for the CPA group, but the differences were small and did not reach statistical significance. The differences may have been related to the antigonadotropic activity of CPA (which would directly counteract the GnRH agonist-induced increase in gonadal androgen production) and/or the fact that bicalutamide requires 4 to 12 weeks of administration to reach steady-state (maximal) levels.

All medically used SAAs are weak partial agonists of the AR rather than silent antagonists, and for this reason, possess inherent androgenicity in addition to their predominantly antiandrogenic actions. In accordance, although CPA produces feminization of and ambiguous genitalia in male fetuses when administered to pregnant animals, it has been found to produce masculinization of the genitalia of female fetuses of pregnant animals. Additionally, all SAAs, including CPA and spironolactone, have been found to stimulate and significantly accelerate the growth of androgen-sensitive tumors in the absence of androgens, whereas NSAAs like flutamide have no effect and can in fact antagonize the stimulation caused by SAAs. Accordingly, unlike NSAAs, the addition of CPA to castration has never been found in any controlled study to prolong survival in prostate cancer to a greater extent than castration alone. In fact, a meta-analysis found that the addition of CPA to castration actually *reduces* the long-term effectiveness of ADT and causes an increase in mortality (mainly due to cardiovascular complications induced by CPA). Also, there is a case report of spironolactone actually inducing *progression* of prostate cancer in a castrated man treated with it for heart failure, and for this reason, spironolactone has been regarded as contraindicated in patients with prostate cancer. Because of their intrinsic capacity to activate the AR, SAAs are incapable of maximally depriving the body of androgen signaling, and will always maintain at least some degree of AR activation.

Due to its progestogenic (and by extension antigonadotropic) activity, CPA is able to suppress circulating testosterone levels by 70–80% in men at high dosages. In contrast,

NSAAs increase testosterone levels by up to 2-fold via blockade of the AR, a difference that is due to their lack of concomitant antigonadotropic action. However, in spite of the combined AR antagonism and marked suppression of androgen levels by CPA (and hence a sort of CAB profile of antiandrogen action), monotherapy with an NSAA, CPA, or a GnRH analogue/castration all have about the same effectiveness in the treatment of prostate cancer, whereas CAB in the form of the addition of bicalutamide (but not of CPA) to castration has slightly but significantly greater comparative effectiveness in slowing the progression of prostate cancer and extending life. These differences may be related to the inherent androgenicity of CPA, which likely serves to limit its clinical efficacy as an antiandrogen in prostate cancer.

Tolerability and Safety

Due to the different hormonal activities of NSAAs like bicalutamide and SAAs like CPA, they possess different profiles of adverse effects. CPA is regarded as having an unfavorable side effect profile, and the tolerability of bicalutamide is considered to be superior. Due to its strong antigonadotropic effects and suppression of androgen and estrogen levels, CPA is associated with severe sexual dysfunction (including loss of libido and impotence) similar to that seen with castration and osteoporosis, whereas such side effects occur little or not at all with NSAAs like bicalutamide. In addition, CPA is associated with coagulation changes and thrombosis (5%), fluid retention (4%), cardiovascular side effects (e.g., ischemic cardiomyopathy) (4–40%), and adverse effects on serum lipid profiles, with severe cardiovascular complications (sometimes being fatal) occurring in approximately 10% of patients. In contrast, bicalutamide and other NSAAs are not associated with these adverse effects. Moreover, CPA has a relatively high rate of generally severe and potentially fatal hepatotoxicity, whereas the risk of hepatotoxicity is far smaller and comparatively minimal with bicalutamide (though not necessarily with other NSAAs, namely flutamide) . CPA has also been associated with high rates of depression (20–30%) and other mental side effects such as fatigue, irritability, anxiety, and suicidal thoughts in both men and women, side effects which may be related to vitamin B12 deficiency.

It has been said that the only advantage of CPA over castration is its relatively low incidence of hot flashes, a benefit that is mediated by its progestogenic activity. Due to increased estrogen levels, bicalutamide and other NSAAs are similarly associated with low rates of hot flashes (9.2% for bicalutamide vs. 5.4% for placebo in the EPC trial). One advantage of CPA over NSAAs is that, because it suppresses estrogen levels rather than increases them, it is associated with only a low rate of what is generally only slight gynecomastia (4–20%), whereas NSAAs are associated with rates of gynecomastia of up to 80%. Although NSAA monotherapy has many tolerability advantages in comparison to CPA, a few of these advantages, such as preservation of sexual function and interest and BMD (i.e., no increased incidence of osteoporosis) and low rates of hot flashes, are lost when NSAAs are combined with castration. However, the risk and severity of gynecomastia with NSAAs are also greatly diminished in this context.

Unlike spironolactone, bicalutamide has no antimineralocorticoid activity, and for this reason, has no risk of hyperkalemia (which can, rarely/in severe cases, result in hospitalization and/or death) or other antimineralocorticoid side effects such as urinary frequency, dehydration, hypotension, hyponatremia, metabolic acidosis, or decreased renal function that may occur with spironolactone treatment.

In women, unlike CPA and spironolactone, bicalutamide does not produce menstrual irregularity or amenorrhea, nor does it interfere with ovulation.

Castration and GnRH Analogues

Castration consists of either medical castration with a GnRH analogue or surgical castration via orchiectomy. GnRH analogues include GnRH agonists like leuprorelin or goserelin and GnRH antagonists like cetrorelix. They are powerful antigonadotropins and work by abolishing the GnRH-induced secretion of gonadotropins, in turn ceasing gonadal production of sex hormones. Medical and surgical castration achieve essentially the same effect, decreasing circulating testosterone levels by approximately 95%.

Effectiveness

Bicalutamide monotherapy has overall been found to be equivalent in effectiveness compared to GnRH analogues and castration in the treatment of prostate cancer. A meta-analysis concluded that there is a slight effectiveness advantage for GnRH analogues/castration, but the differences trend towards but do not reach statistical significance. In mPC, the median survival time was found to be only 6 weeks shorter with bicalutamide monotherapy in comparison to GnRH analogue monotherapy.

Tolerability and Safety

Monotherapy with NSAAs including bicalutamide, flutamide, nilutamide, and enzalutamide shows a significantly lower risk of certain side effects, including hot flashes, depression, fatigue, loss of libido, and decreased sexual activity, relative to treatment with GnRH analogues, CAB (NSAA and GnRH analogue combination), CPA, or surgical castration in prostate cancer. For example, 60% of men reported complete loss of libido with bicalutamide relative to 85% for CAB and 69% reported complete loss of erectile function relative to 93% for CAB. Another large study reported a rate of impotence of only 9.3% with bicalutamide relative to 6.5% for standard care (the controls), a rate of decreased libido of only 3.6% with bicalutamide relative to 1.2% for standard care, and a rate of 9.2% with bicalutamide for hot flashes relative to 5.4% for standard care. One other study reported decreased libido, impotence, and hot flashes in only 3.8%, 16.9%, and 3.1% of bicalutamide-treated patients, respectively, relative to 1.3%, 7.1%, and 3.6% for placebo. It has been proposed that due to the lower relative effect of NSAAs on sexual interest and activity, with two-thirds of advanced mPC patients treated with them retaining sexual interest, these drugs may result in improved quality of life and thus be preferable for those who wish to retain sexual interest and function relative to other antiandrogen therapies in prostate cancer. Also, bicalutamide differs from GnRH analogues (which decrease bone mineral density (BMD) and significantly increase the risk of fractures) in that it has well-documented benefits on BMD, effects that are likely due to increased levels of estrogen.

Cost

Bicalutamide is far less expensive than GnRH analogues, which, in spite of some having been off-patent many years, have been reported (in 2013) to typically cost $10,000 to $15,000 USD per year (or about $1,000 per month) of treatment.

Pharmacology

Antiandrogen

Bicalutamide acts as a highly selective competitive silent antagonist of the AR (IC$_{50}$ = 159–243 nM). It has no capacity to activate the AR under normal physiological circumstances. In addition to competitive antagonism of the AR, bicalutamide has been found to accelerate the degradation of the AR, and this action may also be involved in its activity as an antiandrogen. The activity of bicalutamide lies in the (R)-isomer, which binds to the AR with an affinity that is about 30-fold higher than that of the (S)-isomer. Levels of the (R)-isomer also notably are 100-fold higher than those of the (S)-isomer at steady-state.

Owing to its selectivity for the AR, unlike SAAs such as CPA and megestrol acetate, bicalutamide does not bind to other steroid hormone receptors, and for this reason, has no additional, off-target hormonal activity (estrogenic or antiestrogenic, progestogenic or antiprogestogenic, glucocorticoid or antiglucocorticoid, or mineralocorticoid or antimineralocorticoid); nor does it inhibit 5α-reductase. However, it significantly increases estrogen levels secondary to blockade of the AR in males, and for this reason, does have some *indirect* estrogenic effects in men. Also in contrast to SAAs, bicalutamide neither inhibits nor suppresses androgen production in the body (i.e., it does not act as an antigonadotropin or steroidogenesis inhibitor), and instead exclusively mediates its antiandrogen effects by blocking androgen binding and subsequent receptor activation at the level of the AR.

Drug and Androgen Levels and Efficacy

Although the affinity of bicalutamide for the AR is approximately 50 times lower than that of DHT (IC$_{50}$ ≈ 3.8 nM), the main endogenous ligand of the receptor in the prostate gland, sufficiently high relative concentrations of bicalutamide (1,000-fold excess) are effective in preventing activation of the AR by androgens like DHT and testosterone and subsequent upregulation of the transcription of androgen-responsive genes. At steady-state, relative to the normal adult male range for testosterone levels (300–1,000 ng/dL), circulating concentrations of bicalutamide at 50 mg/day are 600 to 2,500 times higher and at 150 mg/day 1,500 to 8,000 times higher than circulating testosterone levels, while bicalutamide concentrations, relative to the mean testosterone levels present in men who have been surgically castrated (15 ng/dL), are 42,000 times higher than testosterone levels at 50 mg/day.

Whereas testosterone is the major circulating androgen, DHT is the major androgen in the prostate gland. DHT levels in circulation are relatively low and only approximately 10% of those of circulating testosterone levels. Conversely, local concentrations of DHT in the prostate gland are 5- to 10-fold higher than circulating levels of DHT. This is due to high expression of 5α-reductase in the prostate gland, which very efficiently catalyzes the formation of DHT from testosterone such that over 90% of intraprostatic testosterone is converted into DHT. Relative to testosterone, DHT is 2.5- to 10-fold as potent as an AR agonist in bioassays, and hence, is a much stronger androgen in comparison. As such, AR signaling is exceptionally high in the prostate gland, and the effectiveness of bicalutamide monotherapy in the treatment of prostate cancer, which is roughly equivalent to that of GnRH analogues, is a reflection of its capacity to strongly and efficaciously antagonize the AR at clinically used dosages. On the other hand, GnRH analogues achieve only a 50 to 60% reduction in levels of DHT in the prostate gland, and the combination of a GnRH analogue and bicalutamide is significantly more effective than either modality alone in the treatment of prostate cancer.

In women, total testosterone levels are 20-fold and free testosterone levels 40-fold lower relative to men. In addition, whereas bicalutamide monotherapy can increase testosterone levels by up to 2-fold in men, the drug does not increase testosterone levels in women. For these reasons, much lower dosages of bicalutamide (e.g., 25 mg/day in the hirsutism studies) may be used in women with comparable antiandrogen effectiveness.

Influences on Hormone Levels

In men, blockade of the AR by bicalutamide in the pituitary gland and hypothalamus suppresses the negative feedback of androgens on the release of LH, resulting in an elevation in LH levels. Follicle-stimulating hormone (FSH) levels, in contrast, remain essentially unchanged. The increase in LH levels leads to an increase in androgen and estrogen levels. At a dosage of 150 mg/day, bicalutamide has been found to increase testosterone levels by about 1.5- to 2-fold (59–97% increase) and estradiol levels by about 1.5- to 2.5-fold (65–146% increase). Levels of DHT are also increased to a lesser extent (by 25%), and concentrations of sex hormone-binding globulin (SHBG) and prolactin increase as well (by 8% and 40%, respectively) secondary to the increase in estradiol levels. The estradiol concentrations produced by bicalutamide monotherapy in men are said to approximate the low-normal estradiol levels of a premenopausal woman, while testosterone levels generally remain in the high end of the normal male range and rarely exceed it. Dosages of bicalutamide of 10 mg, 30 mg, and 50 mg per day have been found to produce a "moderate" effect on sex hormone levels in men with prostate cancer (notably providing indication that the drug has clinically-relevant antiandrogen effects in males at a dosage as low as 10 mg/day). It is important to note that bicalutamide increases androgen and estrogen levels only in men and not in women; this is because androgen levels are comparatively far lower in women and in turn exert little to no basal suppression of the hypothalamic-pituitary-gonadal (HPG) axis.

The reason that testosterone levels are elevated but almost always remain in the normal male range with bicalutamide monotherapy is thought to be due to the concomitantly increased levels of estradiol, as estradiol is potently antigonadotropic and limits secretion of LH. In fact, estradiol is a much stronger inhibitor of gonadotropin secretion than is testosterone, and even though circulating concentrations of estradiol are far lower than those of testosterone in men, it is said that estradiol is nonetheless likely the major feedback regulator of gonadotropin secretion in this sex. In accordance, clomifene, a SERM with antiestrogenic activity, has been found to increase testosterone levels to as much as 250% of initial values in men with hypogonadism, and a study of clomifene treatment in normal men observed increases in FSH and LH levels of 70–360% and 200–700%, respectively, with increases in testosterone levels that were similar to the increases seen with the gonadotropins. In addition to systemic or circulating estradiol, local aromatization of testosterone into estradiol in the hypothalamus and pituitary gland may contribute to suppression of gonadotropin secretion.

Bicalutamide more than blocks the effects of the increased testosterone levels that it induces in men, which is evidenced by the fact that monotherapy with the drug is about as effective as GnRH analogue therapy in the treatment of prostate cancer. However, in contrast, the effects of the elevated estrogen levels remain unopposed by bicalutamide, and this is largely responsible for the feminizing side effects (e.g., gynecomastia) of the drug in men.

Differences from Castration

It has been proposed that the increase in estrogen levels caused by NSAAs like bicalutamide compensates for androgen blockade in the brain, which may explain differences in the side effect profiles of these drugs relative to GnRH analogues/castration, CAB, and CPA (which, in contrast, decrease both androgen and estrogen levels). In the case of sexual interest and function, this notion is supported by a variety of findings including animal studies showing that estrogen deficiency results in diminished sexual behavior, treatment with tamoxifen resulting in significantly lowered libido in 30% of men receiving it for male breast cancer, and estrogen administration restoring libido and the frequency of sexual intercourse in men with congenital estrogen deficiency, among others.

Several metabolites of testosterone and DHT, including estradiol, 3α-androstanediol, and 3β-androstanediol, are estrogens (mainly potent ERβ agonists in the cases of the latter two), and 3α-androstanediol is additionally a potent $GABA_A$ receptor-potentiating neurosteroid. Due to the fact that bicalutamide does not lower testosterone levels, the levels of these metabolites would not be expected to be lowered either, unlike with therapies such as GnRH analogues. (Indeed, testosterone, DHT, and estradiol levels are actually raised by bicalutamide treatment, and for this reason, levels of 3α- and 3β-androstanediol might be elevated to some degree similarly.) These metabolites of testosterone have been found to have AR-independent positive effects on sexual motivation, and may explain the preservation of sexual interest and function by bicalutamide and other NSAAs. They also have antidepressant, anxiolytic, and cognitive-enhancing effects, and may account for the lower incidence of depression with bicalutamide and other NSAAs relative to other antiandrogen therapies.

Induction of Breast Development

In transgender women, breast development is a desired effect of antiandrogen and/or estrogen treatment. Bicalutamide induces breast development (or gynecomastia) in biologically male individuals by two mechanisms: 1) blocking androgen signaling in breast tissue; and 2) increasing estrogen levels. Estrogen is responsible for the induction of breast development under normal circumstances, while androgens powerfully suppress estrogen-induced breast growth. It has been found that very low levels of estrogen can induce breast development in the presence of low or no androgen signaling. In accordance, bicalutamide not only induces gynecomastia at a high rate when given to men as a monotherapy, it results in a higher incidence of gynecomastia in combination with a GnRH analogue relative to GnRH analogue treatment alone (in spite of the presence of only castrate levels of estrogen in both cases).

A study of men treated with NSAA (flutamide or bicalutamide) monotherapy for prostate cancer found that NSAAs induced full ductal development and moderate lobuloalveolar development of the breasts from a histological standpoint. The study also found that, in contrast, treatment of transgender women with estrogen and CPA (which is progestogenic in addition to antiandrogenic, unlike NSAAs) resulted in full lobuloalevolar development, as well as pregnancy-like breast hyperplasia in two of the subjects. In addition, it was observed that the lobuloalveolar maturation reversed upon discontinuation of CPA after sex reassignment surgery (that is, surgical castration) in these individuals. It was concluded that progestogen in addition to antiandrogen/estrogen treatment is required for the induction of full female-like histological breast development (i.e., that includes complete lobuloalveolar maturation), and that continued progestogen treatment is necessary to maintain such maturation. It should be noted however that although these findings may have important implications in the contexts of lactation and breastfeeding, epithelial tissue accounts for approximately only 10% of breast volume (with the bulk of the breasts (80–90%) being represented by stromal or adipose tissue), and it is uncertain to what extent, if any, that development of lobuloalveolar structures (a form of epithelial tissue) contributes to breast size and/or shape.

Effects on Spermatogenesis and Fertility

Spermatogenesis and male fertility are dependent on FSH, LH, and high levels of intra-testicular testosterone. LH does not seem to be involved in spermatogenesis outside of its role of inducing production of testosterone by the Leydig cells in the seminiferous tubules (which make up approximately 80% of the bulk of the testes), whereas this is not the case for FSH. In accordance with the fact that the testes are the source of 95% of circulating testosterone in the body, levels of testosterone within the testes are extremely high, ranging from 20- to 200-fold higher than circulating concentrations. High levels of intratesticular testosterone are required for spermatogenesis, although only a small fraction (5–10%) of normal intratesticular levels of testosterone appears to actually be necessary for spermatogenesis.

Unlike with antigonadotropic antiandrogens such as CPA and GnRH analogues, it has been reported that bicalutamide monotherapy (at 50 mg/day) has very little effect on the ultrastructure of the testes and on sperm maturation in humans even after long-term therapy (>4 years). This may be explained by the extremely high local levels of testosterone in the testes, in that it is likely that systemic bicalutamide therapy is un-able to produce intratesticular concentrations of the drug that are able to significantly block androgen action in this part of the body. This is particularly so considering that bicalutamide increases circulating testosterone levels, and by extension testicular tes-tosterone production, by up to two-fold in males, and that only a small fraction of nor-mal intratesticular testosterone levels, and by extension androgen action, appears to be necessary to maintain spermatogenesis.

In contrast to bicalutamide and other pure antiandrogens/NSAAs, antigonadotropic antiandrogens suppress gonadotropin secretion, which in turn diminishes testosterone production by the testes as well as the maintenance of the testes by FSH, resulting in at-rophy and loss of their function. As such, bicalutamide and other NSAAs may uniquely have the potential to preserve testicular function and spermatogenesis and thus male fertility relative to alternative therapies. In accordance with this notion, a study found that prolonged, high-dose bicalutamide treatment had minimal effects on fertility in male rats. However, another study found that low-dose bicalutamide administration resulted in testicular atrophy and reduced the germ cell count in the testes of male rats by almost 50%, though the rate of successful fertilization and pregnancy following mating was not assessed.

Treatment of men with exogenous testosterone or other anabolic-androgenic steroids results in suppression of gonadotropin secretion and gonadal testosterone production due to their antigonadotropic effects/activation of the AR in the pituitary gland, result-ing in inhibition or abolition of spermatogenesis and fertility:

Treatment of an infertile man with testosterone does [not] improve spermatogenesis, since exogenous administrated testosterone and its metabolite estrogen will suppress both GnRH production by the hypothalamus and luteinizing hormone production by the pituitary gland and subsequently suppress testicular testosterone production. Also, high levels of testosterone are needed inside the testis and this can never be accomplished by oral or parenteral administration of androgens. Suppression of testosterone production by the leydig cells will result in a deficient spermatogenesis, as can be seen in men taking anabolic-androgenic steroids.

In contrast, pure AR antagonists would, in theory, result in the opposite (although reduced semen volume and sexual dysfunction may occur):

It is theoretically a sound hypothesis that the spermatogenesis can be increased by indirectly stimulating FSH and LH secretions from the pituitary gland. However, for this to fructify, it requires the use of testosterone antagonist to nullify the negative feedback effect of circulating testosterone on the release of FSH and LH, thus augmenting the secretion of testosterone and spermatogenesis. Unfortunately, a testosterone antagonist will be unacceptable to males, as it may reduce secondary sexual functions including erection and ejaculation that is vital for the successful fertilization.

Although bicalutamide alone would appear to have minimal detrimental effect on spermatogenesis and male fertility, other hormonal agents that bicalutamide may be combined with, including GnRH analogues and particularly estrogens (as in transgender hormone therapy), can have a considerable detrimental effect on fertility. This is mainly or completely a consequence of their antigonadotropic activity. Antigonadotropic agents like high-dose CPA, high-dose androgens (e.g., testosterone esters), and GnRH antagonists (though notably not GnRH agonists) produce hypogonadism and high rates of severe or complete infertility (e.g., severe oligospermia or complete azoospermia) in men. However, these effects are fully and often rapidly reversible with their discontinuation, even after prolonged treatment. In contrast, while estrogens at sufficiently high dosages similarly are able to produce hypogonadism and to abolish or severely impair spermatogenesis, this is not necessarily reversible in the case of estrogens and can be long-lasting after prolonged exposure. The difference is attributed to an apparently unique, direct adverse effect of high concentrations of estrogens on the Leydig cells of the testes.

Paradoxical AR activation in Prostate Cancer

Though a pure, or silent antagonist of the AR under normal circumstances, bicalutamide, as well as other earlier antiandrogens like flutamide and nilutamide, have been found to possess weak partial agonist properties in the setting of AR overexpression and agonist activity in the case of certain mutations in the ligand-binding domain of the AR. As both of these circumstances can eventually occur in prostate cancer, resistance to bicalutamide usually develops and the drug has the potential to paradoxically stimulate tumor growth when this happens. This is the mechanism of the phenomenon of antiandrogen withdrawal syndrome, where antiandrogen discontinuation paradoxically slows the rate of tumor growth. The newer drug enzalutamide has been shown not to have agonistic properties in the context of overexpression of the AR, though certain mutations in the AR can still convert it from an antagonist to agonist.

Other Actions

Cytochrome P450 Modulator

It has been reported that bicalutamide may have the potential to inhibit the enzymes CYP3A4 and, to a lesser extent, CYP2C9, CYP2C19, and CYP2D6, based on *in vitro* research. However, no relevant inhibition of CYP3A4 has been observed *in vivo* with bicalutamide at a dose of 150 mg (using midazolam as a specific marker of CYP3A4 activity). In animals, bicalutamide has been found to be an inducer of certain cytochrome P450 enzymes. However, dosages of 150 mg/day or less have shown no evidence of this in humans.

Bicalutamide has been identified as a strong CYP27A1 (cholesterol 27-hydroxylase) inhibitor *in vitro*. CYP27A1 converts cholesterol into 27-hydroxycholesterol, an oxysterol that has multiple biological functions including direct, tissue-specific activation of the estrogen receptor (ER) (it has been characterized as a selective estrogen receptor modulator) and the liver X receptor. 27-Hydroxycholesterol has been found to increase ER-positive breast cancer cell growth via its estrogenic action, and hence, it has been proposed that bicalutamide and other CYP27A1 inhibitors may be effective as adjuvant therapies to aromatase inhibitors in the treatment of ER-positive breast cancer.

Bicalutamide has also been found to bind to and inhibit CYP46A1 (cholesterol 24-hydroxylase) *in vitro*, but this has yet to be assessed and confirmed *in vivo*.

P-Glycoprotein Inhibitor

Bicalutamide, as well as enzalutamide, have been found to act as inhibitors of P-glycoprotein efflux and ATPase activity. This action may reverse docetaxel resistance in prostate cancer cells by reducing transport of the drug out of these cells.

GABA$_A$ Receptor Negative Modulator

All of the NSAAs approved for the treatment of prostate cancer have been found to possess an off-target action of acting as weak non-competitive inhibitors of human GABA$_A$ receptor currents *in vitro* to varying extents. The IC$_{50}$ values are 44 μM for flutamide (as hydroxyflutamide), 21 μM for nilutamide, 5.2 μM for bicalutamide, and 3.6 μM for enzalutamide. In addition, flutamide, nilutamide, and enzalutamide have been found to cause convulsions and/or death in mice at sufficiently high doses. Bicalutamide was notably not found to do this, but this was likely simply due to the limited central nervous system penetration of bicalutamide in this species. In any case, enzalutamide is the only approved NSAA that has been found to be associated with a significantly increased incidence of seizures and other associated side effects clinically, so the relevance of the aforementioned findings with regard to bicalutamide and the other NSAAs is unclear.

Pharmacokinetics

Absorption

Bicalutamide is extensively and well-absorbed following oral administration, and its absorption is not affected by food. The absolute bioavailability of bicalutamide in humans is unknown due to its very low water solubility and hence lack of an assessable intravenous formulation. However, the absolute bioavailability of bicalutamide has been found to be high in animals at low doses (72% in rats at 1 mg/kg; 100% in dogs at 0.1 mg/kg), but diminishes with increasing doses such that the bioavailability of bicalutamide is low at high doses (10% in rats at 250 mg/kg; 31% in dogs at 100 mg/kg). In accordance, absorption of (R)-bicalutamide in humans is slow and extensive but saturable, with steady-state levels increasing linearly at a dosage of up to 50 mg/day and non-linearly at higher dosages. At higher dosages of 100 to 200 mg/day, absorption of bicalutamide is approximately linear, with a small but increasing departure from linearity above 150 mg/day. In terms of geometric mean steady-state concentrations of (R)-bicalutamide, the departures from linearity were 4%, 13%, 17%, and 32% with dosages of 100, 150, 200, and 300 mg/day, respectively. There is a plateau in steady-state levels of (R)-bicalutamide with bicalutamide dosages above 300 mg/day, and, accordingly, dosages of bicalutamide of 300 to 600 mg/day result in similar circulating concentrations of (R)-bicalutamide and similar degrees clinically of efficacy, tolerability, and toxicity. Relative to 150 mg/day bicalutamide, levels of (R)-bicalutamide are about 15% higher at a dosage of 200 mg/day and about 50% higher at a dosage of 300 mg/day. In contrast to (R)-bicalutamide, the inactive enantiomer (S)-bicalutamide is much more rapidly absorbed (as well as cleared from circulation).

Steady-state Concentrations

Pharmacokinetic parameters for bicalut-amide related to circulating concentrations		
	50 mg	**150 mg**
C_{max}	0.77 µg/mL (1.8 µmol/L)	1.4 µg/mL (3.3 µmol/L)
t_{max}	31 hours	39 hours
C_{ss}	8.9 µg/mL (21 µmol/L)	22–28.5 µg/mL (51–66.3 µmol/L)
t_{ss}	4–12 weeks	4–12 weeks
All values are for (R)-bicalutamide		

Steady-state concentrations of the drug are reached after 4 to 12 weeks of administration independently of dosage, with an approximate 10- to 20-fold progressive accumulation of circulating levels of (R)-bicalutamide. In spite of the relatively long time to reach steady-state (which is a product of its long terminal half-life), there is evidence that the achieved AR blockade of bicalutamide is equivalent to that of flutamide by the end of the first day of treatment. With single 50 mg and 150 mg doses of bicalutamide, mean peak concentrations (C_{max}) of (R)-bicalutamide are 0.77 µg/mL (1.8 µmol/L) (at 31 hours) and 1.4 µg/mL (3.3 µmol/L) (at 39 hours), respectively. At steady-state, mean circulating concentrations (C_{ss}) of (R)-bicalutamide with 50 mg/day and 150 mg/day bicalutamide are 8.9 µg/mL (21 µmol/L) and 22 µg/mL (51 µmol/L), respectively. In another 150 mg/day bicalutamide study, mean circulating concentrations of (R)-bicalutamide were 19.4 µg/mL (45.1 µmol/L) and 28.5 µg/mL (66.3 µmol/L) on days 28 and 84 (weeks 4 and 12) of treatment, respectively.

Distribution

The tissue distribution of bicalutamide is not well-characterized. However, it has been reported that distribution studies with bicalutamide have shown that preferential (i.e., tissue-selective) accumulation in anabolic (e.g., muscle) tissues does not occur. There are no available data on hepatic bicalutamide concentrations in humans, but a rat study found that oral bicalutamide treatment resulted in 4-fold higher concentrations of the drug in the liver relative to plasma (a common finding with orally administered drugs, due to transfer through the hepatic portal system prior to reaching circulation). In men receiving 150 mg/day bicalutamide, concentrations of (R)-bicalutamide in semen were 4.9 µg/mL (11 µmol/L), and the amount of the drug that could potentially be delivered to a female partner during sexual intercourse is regarded as low (estimated at 0.3 µg/kg) and below the amount that is required to induce changes in the offspring of laboratory animals. Bicalutamide is highly protein-bound (96.1% for racemic bicalutamide, 99.6% for (R)-bicalutamide), mainly to albumin. It has negligible affinity for SHBG and no affinity for corticosteroid-binding globulin.

Central Penetration

Based on animal research, it was initially thought that bicalutamide was unable to cross the blood-brain-barrier into the central nervous system and hence would be a peripherally-selective antiandrogen in humans. This conclusion was drawn from the finding that bicalutamide does not increase LH or testosterone levels in multiple animal species (including rats and dogs), as antiandrogens like flutamide normally do this by blocking ARs in the pituitary gland and hypothalamus in the brain and thereby disinhibiting the HPG axis. In humans however, bicalutamide has been found to increase LH and testosterone levels, and to a comparative extent relative to flutamide and nilutamide. As such, it appears that there are species differences in the central penetration of bicalutamide and that the drug does indeed cross the blood-brain-barrier and affect central function in humans, as supported by potential side effects, in spite of increased testosterone levels, like hot flashes and diminished sexual interest in men. A newer NSAA, darolutamide, has been found to negligibly cross the blood-brain-barrier in both animals *and* humans, and in accordance, unlike bicalutamide, does not increase LH or testosterone levels in humans.

Metabolism

The metabolism of bicalutamide is hepatic and stereoselective. The inactive (*S*)-enantiomer is metabolized mainly by glucuronidation and is rapidly cleared from circulation, while the active (*R*)-isomer is slowly hydroxylated and glucuronidated. In accordance, the active (*R*)-enantiomer has a far longer half-life than the (*S*)-isomer, and circulating levels of (*R*)-bicalutamide are 10- to 20-fold and 100-fold higher than those of (*S*)-bicalutamide after a single dose and at steady-state, respectively. Bicalutamide is almost exclusively metabolized, via hydroxylation into hydroxybicalutamide, by the cytochrome P450 enzyme CYP3A4. It is also glucuronidated (via UDP-glucuronyltransferase, specifically UGT1A9) into bicalutamide glucuronide, and hydroxybicalutamide glucuronide is formed secondarily from hydroxybicalutamide. Similarly to the inactive (*S*)-enantiomer of bicalutamide, (*R*)-hydroxybicalutamide is glucuronidated and rapidly cleared from circulation. None of the metabolites of bicalutamide are known to be active. Moreover, little, if any of the metabolites are present in circulation, where unchanged bicalutamide predominates. (*R*)-Bicalutamide has a long terminal half-life of 5.8 days with a single dose, and a terminal half-life of 7–10 days with repeated administration, which more than allows for convenient once-daily dosing of bicalutamide.

Elimination

Bicalutamide is eliminated in feces (43%) and urine (34%), whereas its metabolites are eliminated in approximately equal proportions in urine and bile. It is excreted to a substantial extent in its unmetabolized form, with both bicalutamide and its metabolites excreted mainly as glucuronide conjugates.

Variation

The pharmacokinetics of bicalutamide are unaffected by food, age, body weight, renal impairment, and mild-to-moderate hepatic impairment. However, it has been observed that steady-state concentrations of bicalutamide are higher in Japanese individuals than in Caucasians, indicating that ethnicity may be associated with differences in the pharmacokinetics of bicalutamide in some instances.

Chemistry

Chemical Properties

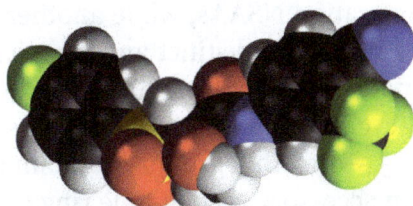

A space-filling model of bicalutamide.

Bicalutamide is a racemic mixture consisting of equal proportions of enantiomers (R)-bicalutamide and (S)-bicalutamide. Its systematic name (IUPAC) is (RS)-N-[4-cyano-3-(trifluoromethyl)phenyl]-3-[(4-fluorophenyl)sulfonyl]-2-hydroxy-2-methylpropanamide. It has a chemical formula of $C_{18}H_{14}F_4N_2O_4S$, a molecular weight of 430.37, and is a fine white to off-white powder. The pKa' of bicalutamide is approximately 12. It is a highly lipophilic compound (log P = 2.92). At 37 °C (98.6 °F), or normal human body temperature, bicalutamide is practically insoluble in water (4.6 mg/L), acid (4.6 mg/L at pH 1), and alkali (3.7 mg/L at pH 8). In organic solvents, it is slightly soluble in chloroform and absolute ethanol, sparingly soluble in methanol, and freely soluble in acetone and tetrahydrofuran.

Structure and Analogues

First-generation NSAAs

First-generation NSAAs including bicalutamide, flutamide, and nilutamide are synthetic, non-steroidal anilide (N-phenylamide) derivatives and structural analogues of each other. Bicalutamide is a diarylpropionamide, while flutamide is a monoarylpropionamide and nilutamide is a hydantoin. Bicalutamide and flutamide, though not nilutamide, can also be classified as toluidides. All three of the compounds share a common 3-trifluoromethylaniline moiety. Bicalutamide is a modification of flutamide in which a 4-fluorophenylsulfonyl moiety has been added and the nitro group on the original phenyl ring has been replaced with a cyano group. Topilutamide, also known as fluridil, is another NSAA that is closely related structurally to the first-generation NSAAs, but, in contrast to them, is not used in the treatment of prostate cancer and is instead used exclusively as a topical antiandrogen in the treatment of androgenic alopecia.

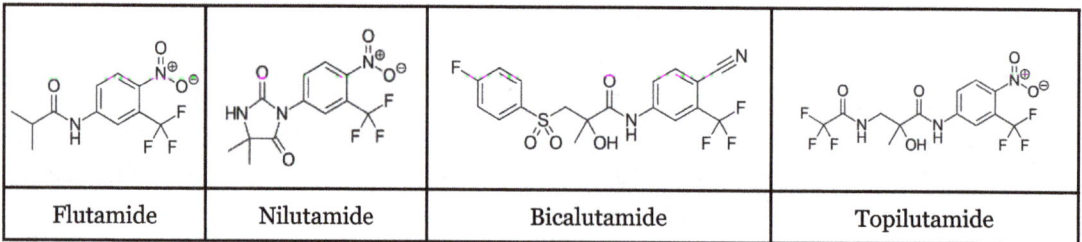

| Flutamide | Nilutamide | Bicalutamide | Topilutamide |

Second-generation NSAAs

The second-generation NSAAs enzalutamide and apalutamide were derived from and are analogues of the first-generation NSAAs, while another second-generation NSAA, darolutamide, is said to be structurally distinct and chemically unrelated to the other NSAAs. Enzalutamide is a modification of bicalutamide in which the inter-ring linking chain has been altered and cyclized into a 5,5-dimethyl-4-oxo-2-thioxoimidazolidine moiety. In apalutamide, the 5,5-dimethyl groups of the imidazolidine ring of enzalutamide are cyclized to form an accessory cyclobutane ring and one of its phenyl rings is replaced with a pyridine ring.

| Enzalutamide | Apalutamide | Darolutamide |

Arylpropionamide SARMs

In 1998, researchers discovered the first non-steroidal androgens (the arylpropio-namides) via structural modification of bicalutamide. Unlike bicalutamide (which is purely antiandrogenic), these compounds show tissue-selective androgenic effects and were classified as selective androgen receptor modulators (SARMs). Lead SARMs of this series included acetothiolutamide, enobosarm (ostarine; S-1), and andarine (acet-amidoxolutamide or androxolutamide; S-4). They are very close to bicalutamide struc-turally, with the key differences being that the linker sulfone of bicalutamide has been replaced with an ether or thioether group to confer agonism of the AR and the 4-fluoro atom of the pertinent phenyl ring has been substituted with an acetamido or cyano group to eliminate reactivity at the position.

| Acetothiolutamide | Enobosarm (ostarine) | Andarine |

Synthesis

A number of chemical syntheses of bicalutamide have been published in the literature.

The first published chemical synthesis of bicalutamide (Tucker et al., 1988) proceeds as follows:

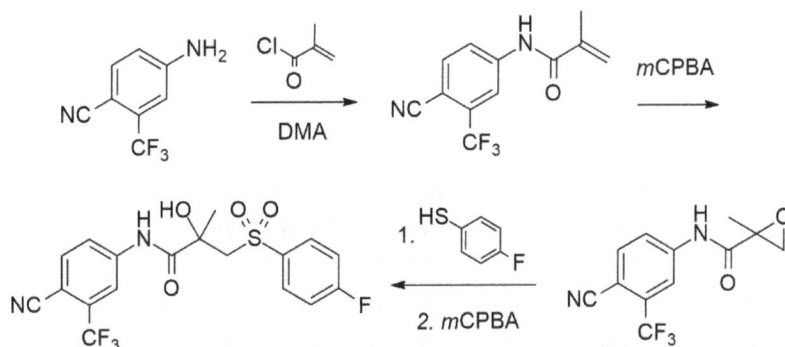

Where the starting material is 4-cyano-3-(trifluoromethyl)aniline (also known as 4-amino-2-(trifluoromethyl)benzonitrile), DMA is dimethylacetamide, and mCPBA is meta-chloroperoxybenzoic acid.

History

All of the marketed NSAAs, including bicalutamide, were derived from flutamide, which was originally synthesized as a bacteriostatic agent in 1967 at Schering Plough Corporation and was subsequently, and serendipitously, found to possess antiandrogen activity. Bicalutamide was discovered by Tucker and colleagues at ICI in the mid-1980s and was selected for development from a group of over 1,000 synthesized compounds. It was first reported in the scientific literature in June 1987, was first studied in a phase I clinical trial in 1987, and the results of the first phase II clinical trial in prostate cancer were published in 1990. In April and May 1995, AstraZeneca began pre-approval marketing of bicalutamide for the treatment of prostate cancer, and it was approved by the U.S. FDA on 4 October 1995 for the treatment of prostate cancer at a dosage of 50 mg/day in combination with a GnRH analogue.

Subsequent to its introduction for use in combination with a GnRH analogue, bicalutamide was developed as a monotherapy at a dosage of 150 mg/day for the treatment of prostate cancer, and was approved for this indication in Europe, Canada, and a number of other countries in the early 2000s. This application of bicalutamide was also under review by the FDA in the U.S. in 2002, but ultimately was not approved in this country. In Japan, bicalutamide is licensed at a dosage of 80 mg/day alone or in combination with a GnRH analogue for prostate cancer. The unique 80 mg dosage of bicalutamide used in Japan was selected for development in this country on the basis of observed pharmacokinetic differences with bicalutamide in Japanese men.

The patent protection of bicalutamide expired in the U.S. in March 2009 and the drug has subsequently been available as a generic, at greatly reduced cost.

Bicalutamide was the fourth antiandrogen (and the third NSAA) to be introduced for the treatment of prostate cancer, following the SAA CPA in 1973 and the NSAAs flutamide and nilutamide in 1975 (1989 in the U.S.) and 1989 (1996 in the U.S.), respectively. It has been followed by abiraterone acetate in 2011 and enzalutamide in 2012, and may also be followed by the in-development drugs apalutamide, darolutamide, galeterone, and seviteronel.

Withdrawal for LPC

In 2003, the EPC trial, comprising over 8,000 patients, reported at 5.4-year follow-up that while 150 mg/day bicalutamide monotherapy increased overall survival in LAPC, it did not increase overall survival in an earlier stage of the disease, LPC (in which the risk of dying from prostate cancer is notably much lower in comparison), and surprisingly, there was, in fact, a trend toward significantly *reduced* overall survival in this group (25.2% death rate for bicalutamide monotherapy versus 20.5% for placebo; hazard ratio = 1.23; 95% confidence interval, 1.00, 1.50). Analyses revealed that bicalutamide monotherapy slightly decreased the rate of mortality due to prostate cancer in this group but accelerated the rate of non-prostate cancer deaths (16.8% for bicalutamide versus 9.5% for placebo). Subsequently, approval for use of bicalutamide monotherapy in this patient population (i.e., LPC) was withdrawn in a number of countries, including the U.K. (in October or November 2003) and several other European countries and Canada (in August 2003), and the U.S. and Canada recommended against the use of 150 mg/day bicalutamide for this indication.

Society and Culture

Generic Name

Bicalutamide is the generic name of bicalutamide in English and the INN, USAN, USP, BAN, DCF, and JAN of the drug. It is also formally referred to as bicalutamidum in Latin, bicalutamida in Spanish and Portuguese, bicalutamid in German, and bikalutamid in Russian and other Slavic languages, whereas its generic name remains unchanged as *bicalutamide* in French.

Bicalutamide is also known by its former developmental code name ICI-176,334.

Brand Names

Bicalutamide is marketed by AstraZeneca in oral tablet form under the brand names Casodex, Cosudex, Calutide, Calumid, and Kalumid in many countries. It is also marketed under the brand names Bicadex, Bicalox, Bicamide, Bicatlon, Bicusan, Binabic, Bypro, Calutol, and Ormandyl among others in various countries. The drug is sold under a large number of generic trade names such as Apo-Bicalutamide, Bicalutamide Accord, Bicalutamide Actavis, Bicalutamide Bluefish, Bicalutamide Kabi, Bicalutamide Sandoz, and Bicalutamide Teva as well. A combination formulation of bicalutamide and goserelin is marketed by AstraZeneca in Australia and New Zealand under the brand name ZolaCos-CP.

Availability

Bicalutamide is available for the treatment of prostate cancer in most developed countries, and is available in at least 70 countries worldwide. For an extensive list of countries in which bicalutamide is marketed along with its corresponding brand names, see here. The drug is registered for use as a 150 mg/day monotherapy for the treatment of LAPC in at least 55 countries, with the U.S. being a notable exception (where it is registered only for use at a dosage of 50 mg/day in combination with castration).

Legal Status

Bicalutamide is a prescription drug. The sale and distribution of prescription drugs is legally regulated throughout much of the world.

Economics

Sales of bicalutamide (as Casodex) in the U.S. were $1.1 billion in 2005, and it has been described as a "billion-dollar-a-year" drug prior to losing its patent protection. In 2014, despite the introduction of abiraterone acetate in 2011 and enzalutamide in 2012, bicalutamide was still the most commonly prescribed drug in the treatment of metastatic castration-resistant prostate cancer (mCRPC). Moreover, in spite of being off-patent, bicalutamide was said to still generate a few hundred million dollars in sales per year for AstraZeneca.

Between January 2007 and December 2009 (a period of three years), 1,232,143 prescriptions were written for bicalutamide in the U.S., or about 400,000 prescriptions per year. During that time, bicalutamide accounted for about 87.2% of the NSAA market, while flutamide accounted for 10.5% of it and nilutamide for 2.3% of it. Approximately 96% of bicalutamide prescriptions were written for diagnosis codes that clearly indicated neoplasm. About 1,200, or 0.1% of bicalutamide prescriptions were dispensed to pediatric patients (age 0–16).

Research

Prostate Cancer

A phase II clinical trial of bicalutamide with everolimus in mCRPC has been conducted.

Bicalutamide has been studied in combination with the 5α-reductase inhibitors finasteride and dutasteride in prostate cancer.

Benign Prostatic Hyperplasia

Bicalutamide has been studied in the treatment of benign prostatic hyperplasia (BPH) in a 24-week trial of 15 patients at a dosage of 50 mg/day. Prostate volume decreased by 26% in patients taking bicalutamide and urinary irritative symptom scores significantly decreased, but peak urine flow rates and urine pressure flow examinations were not significantly different between bicalutamide and placebo. Breast tenderness (93%), gynecomastia (54%), and sexual dysfunction (60%) were all reported as clinically significant side effects at this dosage in these patients, although no treatment discontinuations due to adverse effects occurred and sexual functioning was maintained in 75% of patients.

AR-positive Breast Cancer

Bicalutamide has been tested for the treatment of AR-positive ER/PR-negative locally advanced and metastatic breast cancer in a phase II study for this indication. Enzalutamide may also hold some promise for this type of cancer.

Ovarian Cancer

Bicalutamide has been studied in a phase II clinical trial for ovarian cancer.

Veterinary Use

Bicalutamide is used to treat hyperandrogenism and associated prostatic hyperplasia secondary to hyperadrenocorticism (caused by excessive adrenal androgens) in male ferrets. However, although used, it has not been formally assessed in controlled studies for this purpose.

Neoplasene

Neoplasene is an herbal veterinary medicine derived from certain chemicals, such as sanguinarine, extracted from the perennial herb *Sanguinaria canadensis* (the blood-root plant). It is used to treat cancer in pet animals, especially dogs.Its effectiveness is unproven and there are serious adverse effects.

References

- Plumb, Donald C. (2011). Plumb's Veterinary Drug Handbook, 7th ed. Ames, Iowa: Wiley-Blackwell. pp. 4–5. ISBN 978-0-4709-5965-7.

- Rossi, S, ed. (2013). Australian Medicines Handbook (2013 ed.). Adelaide: The Australian Medicines Handbook Unit Trust. ISBN 978-0-9805790-9-3.

- Joint Formulary Committee (2013). British National Formulary (BNF) (65th ed.). London, UK: Pharmaceutical Press. ISBN 978-0-85711-084-8.

- Brunton, L; Chabner, B; Knollman, B (2010). Goodman and Gilman's The Pharmacological Basis of Therapeutics (12th ed.). New York: McGraw-Hill Professional. ISBN 978-0-07-162442-8.

- Albert Ellis; Gwynn Pennant Ellis (1 January 1987). Progress in Medicinal Chemistry. Elsevier. p. 56. ISBN 978-0-444-80876-9. Retrieved 27 November 2011.

- D. Sriram; P. Yogeeswari (1 September 2010). Medicinal Chemistry. Pearson Education India. p. 299. ISBN 978-81-317-3144-4. Retrieved 27 November 2011.

- Alan F. Schatzberg; Charles B. (2006). Essentials of clinical psychopharmacology. American Psychiatric Pub. p. 7. ISBN 978-1-58562-243-6.

- DiPiro, Joseph T. et al. (2005) Pharmacotherapy: A Pathophysiologic Approach (6th ed.). New York: McGraw-Hill. ISBN 0-07-141613-7.

- Rossi, S, ed. (2013). Australian Medicines Handbook (2013 ed.). Adelaide: The Australian Medicines Handbook Unit Trust. ISBN 978-0-9805790-9-3.

- Taylor, D; Paton, C; Shitij, K (2012). Maudsley Prescribing Guidelines in Psychiatry (11th ed.). West Sussex: Wiley-Blackwell. ISBN 978-0-47-097948-8.

- Lindsay Murray; Frank Daly; David McCoubrie; Mike Cadogan (15 January 2011). Toxicology Handbook. Elsevier Australia. p. 388. ISBN 978-0-7295-3939-5. Retrieved 27 November 2011.

- Dowling PM (February 8, 2005). "Drugs Affecting Appetite". In Kahn CM, Line S, Aiello SE. The Merck Veterinary Manual (9th ed.). John Wiley & Sons. ISBN 0-911910-50-6. Retrieved on October 26, 2008.

5

Veterinary Procedures: An Integrated Study

Animal euthanasia is the act of putting an animal to death. The usual reasons for euthanasia are incurable diseases or unfortunately the lack of resources. Alternatively, the other veterinary procedures mentioned are dysthanasia, organ replacement in animals, tibial tuberosity advancement and an overview of discretionary invasive procedures on animals. This chapter will provide an integrated understanding of veterinary procedures.

Animal Euthanasia

Animal euthanasia is the act of putting an animal to death or allowing it to die by withholding extreme medical measures. Reasons for euthanasia include incurable (and especially painful) conditions or diseases, lack of resources to continue supporting the animal, or laboratory test procedures. Euthanasia methods are designed to cause minimal pain and distress. Euthanasia is distinct from animal slaughter and pest control although in some cases the procedure is the same.

In domesticated animals, this process is commonly referred to by euphemisms such as "put down", "put to sleep", or "put out of his/her/its misery".

Methods

The methods of anesthesia can be divided into pharmacological and physical methods. Acceptable pharmacological methods include injected drugs and gases that first depress the central nervous system and then cardiovascular activity. Acceptable physical methods must first cause rapid loss of consciousness by disrupting the central nervous system. The most common methods are discussed here, but there are other acceptable methods used in different situations.

Intravenous Anesthetic

Unconsciousness, respiratory then cardiac arrest follow rapidly, usually within 30 seconds. Observers generally describe the method as leading to a quick and peaceful death.

For companion animals euthanized in animal shelters, 14 states in the US now prescribe intravenous injection as the required method. These laws date to 1990, when

Georgia's "Humane Euthanasia Act" became the first state law to mandate this method. Before that, gas chambers and other means were commonly employed. The Georgia law was resisted by the Georgia Commissioner of Agriculture, Tommy Irvin, who was charged with enforcing the act. In March 2007, he was sued by former State Representative Chesley V. Morton, who wrote the law, and subsequently ordered by the Court to enforce all provisions of the Act.

Some veterinarians perform a two-stage process: an initial injection that simply renders the pet unconscious and a second shot that causes death. This allows the owner the chance to say goodbye to a live pet without their emotions stressing the pet. It also greatly mitigates any tendency toward spasm and other involuntary movement which tends to increase the emotional upset that the pet's owner experiences.

For large animals, the volumes of barbiturates required are considered by some to be impractical, although this is standard practice in the United States. For horses and cattle, other drugs may be available. Some specially formulated combination products are available, such as Somulose (Secobarbital/Cinchocaine) and Tributame (Embutramide/Chloroquine/Lidocaine), which cause deep unconsciousness and cardiac arrest independently with a lower volume of injection, thus making the process faster, safer, and more effective.

Occasionally, a horse injected with these mixtures may display apparent seizure activity before death. This may be due to premature cardiac arrest. However, if normal precautions (e.g., sedation with detomidine) are taken, this is rarely a problem. Anecdotal reports that long term use of phenylbutazone increase the risk of this reaction are unverified.

After the animal has expired, it is not uncommon for the body to have posthumous body jerks, or for the animal to have a sudden bladder outburst.

Inhalants

Gas anesthetics such as isoflurane and sevoflurane can be used for euthanasia of very small animals. The animals are placed in sealed chambers where high levels of anesthetic gas are introduced. Death may also be caused using carbon dioxide once unconsciousness has been achieved by inhaled anaesthetic. Carbon dioxide is often used on its own for euthanasia of wild animals. There are mixed opinions on whether it causes distress when used on its own, with human experiments lending support to the evidence that it can cause distress and equivocal results in non-humans. In 2013, the American Veterinary Medical Association (AVMA) issued new guidelines for carbon dioxide induction, stating that a flow rate of 10% to 30% volume/min is optimal for the humane euthanization of small rodents.

Carbon monoxide is often used, but some states in the US have banned its use in animal shelters: although carbon monoxide poisoning is not particularly painful, the conditions in the gas chamber are often not humane. Nitrogen has been shown to be effective, although some young animals are rather resistant and it currently is not widely used.

Cervical Dislocation

Cervical dislocation, or displacement of the neck, is an older yet less common method of killing small animals such as mice. Performed properly it is intended to cause as painless death as possible and has no cost or equipment involved. The handler must know the proper method of executing the movement which will cause the cervical displacement and without proper training and method education there is a risk of not causing death and can cause severe pain and suffering. It is unknown how long an animal remains conscious, or the level of suffering it goes through after a correct snapping of the neck, which is why it has become less common and often substituted with inhalants.

Intracardiac or Intraperitoneal Injection

When intravenous injection is not possible, euthanasia drugs such as pentobarbital can be injected directly into a heart chamber or body cavity.

While intraperitoneal injection is fully acceptable (although it may take up to 15 minutes to take effect in dogs and cats), an intracardiac (IC) injection may only be performed on an unconscious or deeply sedated animal. Performing IC injections on a fully conscious animal in places with humane laws for animal handling is often a criminal offense.

Shooting

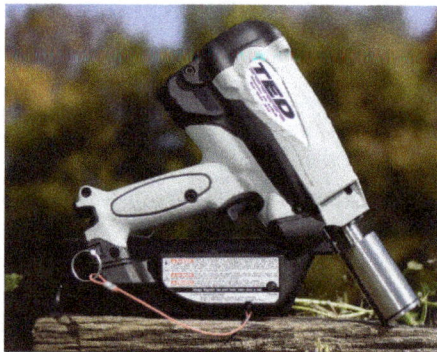

Captive bolt device

This can be an appropriate means of euthanasia for large animals (e.g., horses, cattle, deer) if performed properly. This may be performed by means of:

Free bullet

Traditionally used for shooting horses. The horse is shot in the forehead with the bullet directed down the spine through the medulla oblongata, resulting in instant death. The risks are minimal if carried out by skilled personnel in a suitable location.

Captive bolt

Commonly used for cattle and other livestock. The bolt is fired through the fore-head causing massive disruption of the cerebral cortex. In cattle, this stuns the animal, though if left for a prolonged period it will die from cerebral oedema. Death should therefore be rapidly brought about by pithing or exsanguination. Horses are killed outright by the captive bolt, making pithing and exsanguination unnecessary.

Reasons for Euthanasia

The reasons for euthanasia of pets and other animals include:

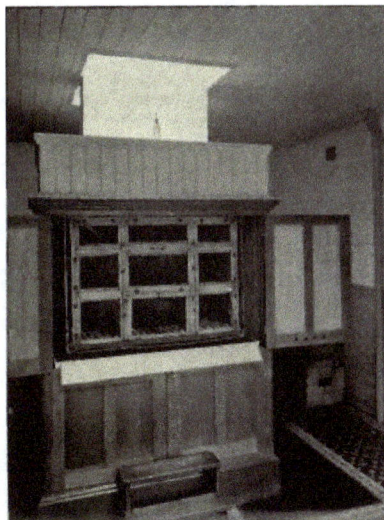

Lethal chamber in the Royal London Institute and Home for Lost and Starving Cats

- Terminal illness, e.g. cancer or rabies

- Illness or accident that is not terminal but would cause suffering for the animal to live with, or when the owner cannot afford, or when the owner has a moral objection to the treatment

- Behavioral problems (usually ones that cannot be corrected) e.g. aggression - Canines that have usually caused grievous bodily harm to either humans or other animals through mauling are usually seized and euthanized ('destroyed' in British legal terms).

- Old age and deterioration leading to loss of major bodily functions, resulting in severe impairment of the quality of life

- Lack of home or caretaker

- Research and testing – In the course of scientific research or testing, animals may be euthanized in order to be dissected, to prevent suffering after testing, to prevent the spread of disease, or other reasons.

Small animal euthanasia is typically performed in a veterinary clinic or hospital or in an animal shelter and is usually carried out by a veterinarian or a veterinary technician working under the veterinarian's supervision. Often animal shelter workers are trained to perform euthanasia as well. Some veterinarians will perform euthanasia at the pet owner's home—this is virtually mandatory in the case of large animal euthanasia. In the case of large animals which have sustained injuries, this will also occur at the site of the accident, for example, on a racecourse.

Some animal rights organizations support animal euthanasia in certain circumstances and practice euthanasia at shelters that they operate.

Remains

Many pet owners choose to have their pets cremated or buried after the pet is euthanized, and there are pet funeral homes that specialize in animal burial or cremation. Otherwise, the animal facility will often freeze the body and subsequently send it to the local landfill.

In some instances, animals euthanized at shelters or animal control agencies have been sent to meat rendering facilities to be processed for use in cosmetics, fertilizer, gelatin, poultry feed, pharmaceuticals and pet food. It was proposed that the presence of pento-barbital in dog food may have caused dogs to become less responsive to the drug when being euthanized. However, a 2002 FDA study found no dog or cat DNA in the foods they tested, so it was theorized that the drug found in dog food came from euthanized cattle and horses. Furthermore, the level of the drug found in pet food was safe.

Dysthanasia (Animal)

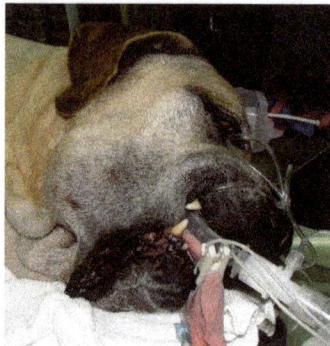

A geriatric mastiff with multiple tumors is being prepared for palliative surgery.

Animal dysthanasia refers to the practice of prolonging the life of animals that are seriously or even terminally ill and that are potentially experiencing suffering. Animal dysthanasia is a recent concept, emerging from changes in the social perception of animals and from advances in veterinary care.

Context

Animal dysthanasia is particularly relevant in the context of small animal practice. For centuries, domestic animals in Western societies used to be mainly farm animals. With the industrialization process, humans become increasingly concentrated in urban areas, having preferential contact with companion animals, namely cats and dogs. While farm animals are widely seen as property, companion animals are perceived as family members with whom humans keep close bonds and develop strong emotional relationships.

At the same time, scientific advances in the field of veterinary medicine enable practitioners to reach accurate diagnoses faster and more reliably than before, allowing life-threatening illnesses to be identified in the early stages of their development. In addition, more advanced options of treatment are currently available which may sometimes be used to prolong the lives of animals as much as possible regardless of their quality.

Causes

Decision upon animal euthanasia often takes into account the relief of pain and suffering. Animal dysthanasia occurs because there is no agreement upon the acceptable and recognizable endpoints of the lives of companion animals. This is due to several reasons. The keeper (guardian; owner) may wish to extend the animal's life because he rejects euthanasia as an acceptable solution. On the other hand, the veterinarian may have a scientific interest on studying the progress of a specific illness or even a financial interest in keeping the patient alive. The keeper and the veterinarian may also want to make use of all possible treatment resources before making the decision of euthanasia. Genuine belief on the animal's recovery and emotional attachment can also interfere on the decision-making process of euthanasia. Situations like these can be especially problematic in some veterinary specialities like small animal oncology where the course of the disease may be difficult to predict and the treatments themselves can cause severe distress.

Organ Replacement in Animals

When an animal experiences organ failure, organ replacement therapies can be used to treat diseased or injured pets. Veterinarians can use many of the same types of therapies that are used in human medicine.

Total Hip Replacement

A good candidate for total hip replacement (THR) must be at least 9–12 months old to be sure he has finished developing and weigh at least 30 lb. The hip implant for dogs is similar to its human counterpart, but it is much smaller. X-rays are used to determine the dimensions of an appropriately sized implant.

The femoral stem is usually made of cobalt chrome or stainless steel, while the cup is made of ultra high molecular weight polyethylene. Polymethyl methacrylate is the cement used with cemented implants, whereas 250-micrometres (diameter) titanium beads usually cover the stem surface of the press-fit implants.

The THR is expected to last 10–15 years, which usually surpasses the remaining life-time of the dog. In less than 5% of cases, the THR will malfunction through loosening of the acetabular cup or femoral fracture. However rare these failures are, they must be corrected immediately with revision surgery.

Pacemaker Implants

The first pacemaker surgery on a dog was performed in 1968. About 300 pacemakers are implanted in dogs each year, even though about 4000 dogs are in need of one. There are no pacemakers made specifically for use in dogs, but human pacemaker users are often outlasted by their pacemakers, leaving behind a functioning pacemaker with less battery power left than a new pacemaker which could be implanted into a dog. One difficulty in implanting used pacemakers is the removal from the deceased human - the pacemaker leads often experience accumulation of surrounding heart muscle tissue and become difficult to remove after death. If the leads are cut in order to remove the pacemaker donation is not possible. If a pacemaker has not been used by a human but has reached its expiry date it will not be suitable for use in a human but could still be used in a dog.

Blood Transfusion

For a blood transfusion to take place, the donor and recipient must be of compatible blood types. Dogs have eleven blood types but are born without antibodies in their blood. For this reason, first time transfusions will not have a reaction, but further transfusions will cause severe reactions if the dog has a mismatch in the DEA1.1 blood type. Because the immune systems of dogs are so fierce, cross-match tests must be per-formed upon each dog blood transfusion. Only about one in every 15 dogs is negative for all antigens and thus, a universal donor. Cats have A, B, and AB blood types with specific factors, but there is no universal donor type Recipient and donor blood must be properly cross-matched. Red cells from the donor are mixed with the serum of the recipient in major cross-matching. In a minor cross-match, the recipient's red cells are compared with the donor's serum. Blood donors must meet specific requirements in order to qualify to donate. They must weigh at least 50 lb for dogs and 10 lb for cats, have high enough blood component values, and have no infectious diseases. One donation could be used by up to two animals.

Policy regarding how donor animals are treated varies. In April, 2014, a veterinarian office in Fort Worth Texas, was accused of keeping dogs that had been presumed to have been euthanized, and using the animals for blood withdrawal.

Heart Valves

Open-heart surgery for dogs requires a six- to eight-person team to carefully monitor the patient before and during the invasive surgery. The entire surgery lasts five hours, during which time the dog is connected to a blood oxygenator and the heart is bypassed. The defective heart valve is removed and the replacement valve, typically from bovine pericardium, is precisely sewn into place. The dog's heart is then restarted and monitored for at least two hours after the surgery is completed. Due to the expense, this is not a common procedure.

Prosthetic Limbs

While small dogs and cats can survive comfortably with three legs, larger dogs, horses, and farm animals require the limb to support their weight. Surgery has also been done on birds that are used for breeding purposes. Each prosthetic limb is custom-made to fit the individual needs of the specific animal.

Orthopedic Implants

UC Davis' equine orthopedic surgery program has developed an implant that has been successful in human surgery for a long time. The intermedullary interlocking nail is used to treat horses with long leg bone fractures. The nails are positioned within the medullary cavity and can be secured to the proximal and distal fracture segments using transcortical screws which penetrate both cortices of the bone, as well as pass through holes in the nail. The nail is placed centrally in the axis of the bone to give full support unlike bone plates that only give exterior support. In an attempt to aid horses with bowed tendons, research has been done using carbon fiber implants that consist of about 40,000 fibers in total each of which is 8 micrometres in diameter. These fibers induce tissue growth and result in a structure of carbon and tissue about 8 mm in diameter.

Tibial Tuberosity Advancement

Tibial Tuberosity Advancement (TTA) is an orthopedic procedure to repair deficient cranial cruciate ligaments in dogs. It has also been used in cats. This procedure was developed by Dr. Slobodan Tepic and Professor Pierre Montavon at the School of Veterinary Medicine, University of Zurich, in Zurich, Switzerland beginning in the late 1990s.

The cranial cruciate ligament (CrCL) in dogs, provides the same function as the anterior cruciate ligament in humans. It stabilizes the knee joint, called the stifle joint in quadrupeds, and limits the tibia from sliding forward in relation to the femur. It is attached to the cranial (anterior) medial side of the interdylar notch of the tibia at one end and the caudal (posterior) side of the lateral femoral condyle at the other end. It also helps to prevent the stifle (knee) joint from over-extending or rotating.

Trauma to the equivalent ligament in humans is common, and damage most frequently occurs during some form of sporting activity (including football, rugby and golf). The nature of the injury is very different in dogs. Rather than the ligament suddenly breaking due to excessive trauma, it usually degenerates slowly over time, rather like a fraying rope. This important difference is the primary reason why the treatment options recommended for cruciate ligament injury in dogs are so different from the treatment options recommended for humans.

In the vast majority of dogs, the cranial cruciate ligament (CrCL) ruptures as a result of long-term degeneration, whereby the fibres within the ligament weaken over time. We do not know the precise cause of this, but genetic factors are probably most important, with certain breeds being predisposed (including Labradors, Rottweilers, Boxers, West Highland White Terriers and Newfoundlands). Supporting evidence for a genetic cause was primarily obtained by assessment of family lines, coupled with the knowledge that many animals will rupture the CrCL in both knees, often relatively early in life. Other factors such as obesity, individual conformation, hormonal imbalance and certain inflammatory conditions of the joint may also play a role. Uncorrected CrCL deficiencies have been associated with meniscal damage and degenerative joint diseases such as osteoarthritis.

TTA is a surgical procedure designed to correct CrCL deficient stifles. The objective of the TTA is to advance the tibial tuberosity, which changes the angle of the patellar ligament to neutralize the tibiofemoral shear force during weight bearing. A microsaggital saw is used to cut the Tibial Tuberosity off then a special titanium cage is used to advance the tibial tuberosity. A titanium plate is used to hold the tibial tuberosity in position. By neutralizing the shear forces in the stifle caused by a ruptured or weakened CrCL, the joint becomes more stable without compromising joint congruency.

TTA appears to be a less invasive procedure than some other techniques for stabilizing the deficient cranial cruciate ligament such as TPLO (Tibial Plateau Leveling Osteotomy) and TWO (Tibial Wedge Osteotomy), as TTA does not disrupt the primary loading axis of the tibia.

Recently, TR BioSurgical has developed a bioscaffold to be used for veterinary osteotomies as a substitute for autologous cancellous bone grafting.

In 2012 TTA RAPID was introduced by the German manufacturer RITA LEIBINGER Medical GmbH & Co. KG in cooperation with the University of Ghent, Belgium. The TTA RAPID implant is a biocompatible sponge-construction which combines a wedge-cage with a plate on the top. In this way there is only one implant needed for the whole TTA surgery. It is called "rapid" because the implantation is very quick, easy to learn and offers a high stability. The surgery is based on the Maquet-Hole-Technique.

Overview of Discretionary Invasive Procedures on Animals

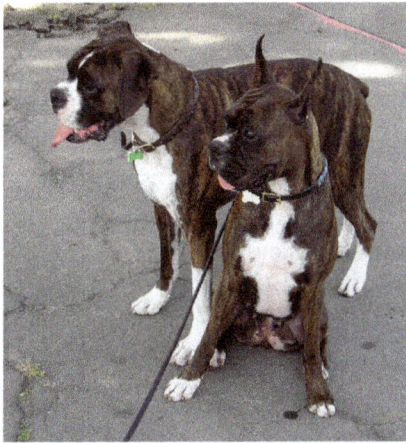

Boxers with natural and cropped ears and docked tails

Numerous procedures performed on domestic animals are more invasive than purely cosmetic alterations, but differ from types of veterinary surgery that are performed exclusively for urgent health reasons. Such procedures have been grouped together under the technical term "mutilatory" by the Royal College of Veterinary Surgeons in a report describing the reasons for their being conducted and their welfare consequences, and by others.

The term "mutilatory" generally connotes some form of disfigurement or even maiming. However, there are multiple definitions and interpretations that carry varying degrees of emotional intensity. For example, Merriam-Webster defines "mutilate" as "to cut up or alter radically so as to make imperfect", but gives a relatively mild example: "the child mutilated the book with his scissors". Thus, while the Royal College of Veterinary Surgeons noted that the term "mutilation" is often an emotive one, having implications in common usage of maiming and disfigurement, they stated that there was no satisfactory alternative term that would suffice for their purposes. Their definition is a narrower one: "covering all procedures, carried out with or without instruments which involve interference with the sensitive tissues or the bone structure of an animal, and are carried out for non-therapeutic reasons."

The following table contains procedures performed on domesticated animals that may or may not have a purported therapeutic purpose.

Invasive procedures on animals	
Species	**Procedures**
Cats	• Claw removal • Devocalization • Tattoo • Tendonectomy
Cattle	• Branding • Dehorning • Ear tagging • Nose ringing • Tongue resection (calves)
Dogs	• Devocalization/Debarking • Dewclaw removal • Ear cropping • Tail docking • Eyelid tacking[a] • Tail nicking[b] • Tattooing • Teeth removal
Ferrets	• De-scenting[c] • Tattooing
Horses	• Branding • Pin firing[d] • Tail blocking[e] • Tail docking • Tail nicking[f]
Laboratory mice	• Ear tagging • Ear notching • Tail clipping[g] • Tattooing • Toe clipping[h]

Pigs	• Ear docking • Ear tagging • Ear notching • Nose ringing • Tail docking • Tattooing • Teeth cutting • Tusk trimming
Poultry	• Beak-trimming • Blinders[i] • Desnooding[j] • Detoeing • Devoicing • Dewinging • Dubbing[k] • Pinioning[l] • Spur removal • Toe clipping
Sheep	• Ear tagging • Ear notching • Dehorning • Marking[m] • Mulesing[n] • Tail docking • Teeth grinding
Skunks	• De-scenting
Prawns/Shrimp	• Eyestalk ablation[o]
Various[p]	• Castration/(caponization) • Earmarking • Ear tagging • Tattooing

References

- Mitchell, Mark A.; Tully, Thomas N. (2009). Manual of exotic pet practice. Elsevier Health Sciences. p. 372. ISBN 978-1-4160-0119-5.

- Villeda, Ray (2014-04-29). "Fort Worth Vet Accused of Keeping Dog Alive for Transfusions | NBC 5 Dallas-Fort Worth". Nbcdfw.com. Retrieved 2016-01-03.

- "What Do Animal Shelters Do with the Bodies of Dead Pets?". Knoji: Consumer Knowledge. 21 February 2011. Retrieved May 21, 2014.

- "Animal Rights Uncompromised:'No-Kill' Shelters", PETA, Retrieved 26 June 2010; "A reply from PETA to a letter inquiring about its euthanization decisions", Petrescueonline.net, Retrieved 26 June 2010.

- Allen, Moira Anderson (2002). "The Final Farewell: How to Handle a Pet's Remains". Pet Loss Support Page. Retrieved 9 June 2010.

- Porstner, Donna (15 April 2004). "Pet funeral home offers services for grieving owners". Boston. com. Retrieved 9 June 2010.

- Becker, Geoffrey S. (17 March 2004). "Animal Rendering: Economics and Policy" (PDF). The National Agricultural Law Centre: Congressional Research Service Reports. Retrieved 9 June 2010.

- "Chapter 9, Food and Agricultural Industries" (PDF). Compilation of Air Pollutant Emission Factors. Retrieved 9 June 2010.

- Myers, Michael (2004). "CVM Scientists Develop PCR Test to Determine Source of Animal Products in Feed, Pet Food". FDA Veterinarian Newsletter. XIX (1). Retrieved 8 June 2010.

- "Report on the risk from pentobarbital in dog food". US Food and Drug Administration. 28 February 2002. Archived from the original on 30 April 2008. Retrieved 9 June 2010.

6

Cosmetic Procedures on Animals

Onychectomy is the process of surgically declawing any animal. The claw bone is amputated because it develops germinal tissue. This act is practiced in some countries whereas in some countries it is considered to be an act of animal cruelty. The other cosmetic procedures that are performed on animals are docking, cropping and devocalization. The major categories of cosmetic procedures are dealt with great details in the chapter.

Onychectomy

Onychectomy, popularly known as declawing, is an operation to remove an animal's claws surgically by means of the amputation of all or part of the distal phalanges, or end bones, of the animal's toes. Because the claw develops from germinal tissue within the third phalanx, amputation of the bone is necessary to fully remove the claw. The terms "onychectomy" and "declawing" imply mere claw removal, but a more appropriate description would be phalangectomy, excision of toe bone.

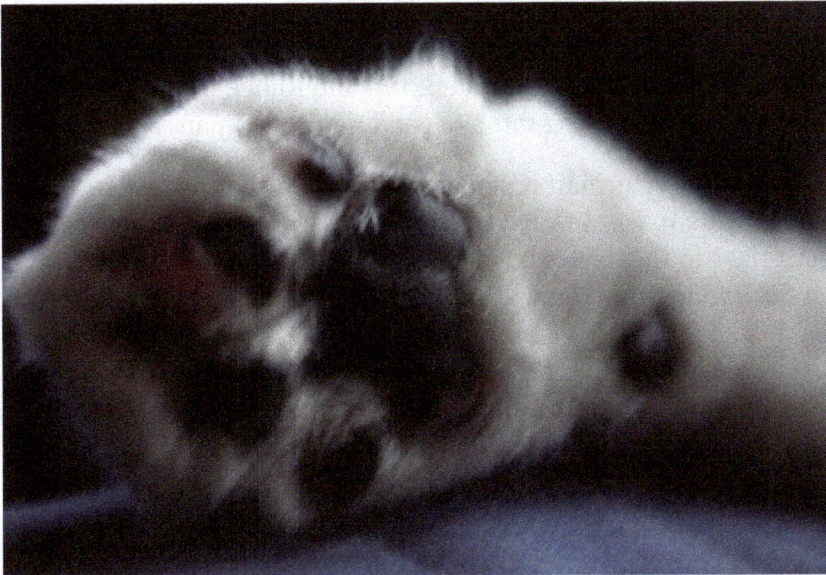

Close-up of a declawed paw.

Although common in North America, declawing is considered an act of animal cruelty in many countries.

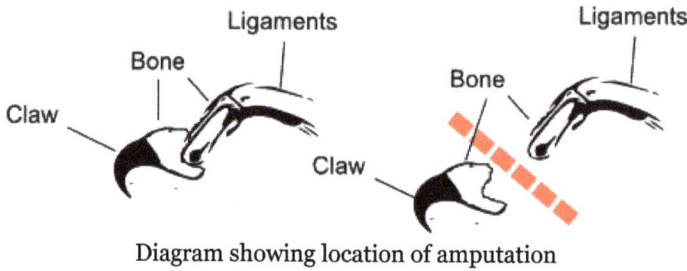

Diagram showing location of amputation

Medically Indicated Onychectomy

The amputation of the distal phalanx is indicated in case of chronic inflammatory processes, tumours, persistent and severe infections and gangrene that are limited to the distal phalanx. The procedure is usually limited to the affected claw, leaving the healthy claws (if any) intact.

Elective Onychectomy

In North America, declawing is commonly performed on cats to prevent damage to household possessions by scratching and to prevent scratching of people. The surgery involves amputating the distal phalanges of all toes on the front paws, and sometimes the rear paws as well. Although no precise figures are available, peer-reviewed veterinary journal articles estimate that approximately 25% of domestic cats in North America have been declawed. Some privately owned apartment buildings in the U.S. ban cats unless they have been declawed. This is not the case in publicly subsidized housing, however, because in 2007 the U.S. Congress enacted legislation that forbids public housing authorities from having such rules. Laws have been passed in California (2012) and Rhode Island (2013) that ban landlords from requiring the declawing cats as a condition of occupancy.

Some North American veterinarians hold the position that people with compromised immune systems, due to conditions such as AIDS, should have their cats declawed to prevent health risks to themselves. However, the U.S. Centers for Disease Control advises against declawing, even in the case of FIV, as "cats need their claws for a number of activities." Instead, the CDC recommends that those with HIV should avoid situations where they might get scratched. Similarly, the National Institutes of Health (NIH) suggests avoiding rough play. As a precautionary measure, *Familydoctor.org* advises people should avoiding provoking cats into scratching them.

Methods

Despite the prevalence of elective onychectomy in North America, no standard practices exist regarding the surgical techniques or surgical tools used, the administration of post-operative analgesics or other follow-up care, or the optimal age or other attributes of cats undergoing the procedure. There are three surgical methods: scalpel blade, guillotine trimmers, and laser.

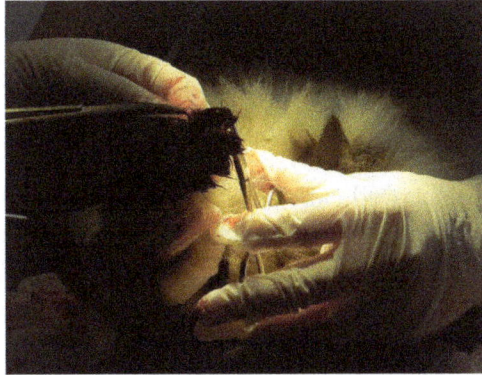

Onychectomy being performed

Recovery, Health and Behavioral Effects

Onychectomy is an orthopedic surgery involving 1 (or more) separate phalangeal amputations, which requires general anesthesia and multi-modal pain management before, during, and after surgery.

In a survey of 276 cat owners, 34% reported post-surgical discomfort in their cats while 78% reported primarily tenderness. Recovery time took from three days to two weeks. Increased biting strength or frequency was reported in 4% of cats, but overall, 96% of owners were satisfied with the surgery. Some other studies found lameness after onychectomy lasting >3 days, >1 week, 8 days, > 12 days, 180 days, and 96 months.

At one veterinary teaching hospital, between 50 and 80% of cats had one or more medical complications post-surgery; 19.8% developed complications after release. Other studies have reported medical post-op complication rates as 24% (Jankowski 1998), 53% (Martinez 1993), 1.4% (Pollari 1996), 82.5% for blade and 51.5% for shear technique (Tobias 1994), and 80% (Yeon 2001). Reported medical complications include: pain, hemorrhage, laceration of paw pads, swelling, reluctance to bear weight on affected limb, neuropraxia (transient motor paralysis), radial nerve damage, lameness, infection, abscess, tissue necrosis, wound dehiscence, incomplete healing, protrusion of 2nd (middle) phalanx, claw regrowth, scurs (growth of deformed claw segments), retention of flexor process of third phalanx, chronic draining tracts, self-mutilation, dermatitis, lethargy, palmigrade stance (walking on wrists), chronic intermittent lameness, chronic pain syndrome, flexor tendon contracture, and cystitis (stress-associated bladder inflammation). Claw regrowth has been seen by veterinarians anywhere from weeks up to 15 years after onychectomy.(Veterinary Information Network).

In post-operation follow ups Yeon, et al. (2001) found six of thirty-nine cats (15%~) were house soiling and seven (18%) had increased biting frequency or intensity. The authors concluded based on this and previous studies that "behavioral problems following onychectomy were not pronounced". Follow-ups in this study were conducted an average of eleven and a half months after surgery.

Behavior problems are a primary cause of cats being relinquished to shelters. Proponents of declawing argue that declawing reduces undesired behaviors (scratching) and thus reduces the likelihood of relinquishment. Opponents of declawing argue the surgery itself creates more behavioral problems leading to relinquishment of cats. A study by Patronek et al. (1996) found in a univariate analysis that declawed cats were only 63% as likely to be relinquished as non-declawed cats. A multivariate analysis conducted in the same study shows odds of being relinquished to a shelter were 89% higher for declawed cats. The authors concluded that the conflicting results of the two analysis made it difficult to interpret the effects of declawing. In a shelter setting, more declawed cats were reported by their owners to have problems with inappropriate elimination (house soiling). However, this study ultimately found no association between the declaw status of cats and their aggression towards humans or frequency of inappropriate elimination (house soiling).

In another study, 16% of declawed cats developed behavior problems (12% biting), and more declawed (55%) than clawed (45%) cats were referred to a vet teaching hospital for behavior problems. This was the second-longest follow-up period (2 years) ever examined.

Patronek, Glickman and Beck (1996) found no association between the declaw status of cats and the frequency of inappropriate elimination (house soiling).

In another study of 275 cats, 11 cats (4%) developed or had worse behavior problems post-declawing; 5 clients (less than 1%) reported that their cats had developed litterbox and biting problems.

Chronic pain syndrome of onychectomy has been described by a pain management specialist as leading to unwanted behaviors, including increased aggression.

A prospective study comparing declawing with tendonectomy noted many medical as well as behavior complications.

An internet survey found that declawed cats were more likely to jump on tables and counters and house-soiled more than non-declawed cats (25% vs. 15%).

However, the current (2009) American Veterinary Medical Association (AVMA) policy statement on declawing states: "There is no scientific evidence that declawing leads to behavioral abnormalities when the behavior of declawed cats is compared with that of cats in control groups."

Declawing Practices

Laws and policies governing onychectomy vary around the world. For example, many European countries prohibit or significantly restrict the practice, as do Australia, New Zealand, Japan, and Turkey. It is banned in at least 22 countries. The list below gives an overview of the situation in different parts of the world.

Australia

In Australia, declawing has never been common, and for all practical purpose, does not exist. Nationwide legislation was recently enacted that prohibits the declawing of cats except for medical need of the cat. The Australian Veterinary Association's policy states: "Surgical alteration to the natural state of an animal is acceptable only if it is necessary for the health and welfare of the animal concerned. Performance of any surgical procedure for other than legitimate medical reasons is unacceptable."

Brazil

In Brazil, declawing is not allowed by the Federal Council of Veterinary Medicine.

Israel

In Israel, the Knesset Education Committee voted unanimously to send a bill banning the declawing of cats not for medical reasons. The bill has passed second and third readings on November 28, 2011, effectively making declawing a criminal offense with penalty of 1 year in prison or a fine of 75,000 Shekels.

Europe

In many European countries the practice is forbidden either under the terms of the European Convention for the Protection of Pet Animals or under Local Animal Abuse Laws, unless it is for "veterinary medical reasons or for the benefit of any particular animal." Some European countries go further, such as Finland, Sweden, Estonia, the Netherlands, Germany and Switzerland, where declawing cats for non-medical reasons is always illegal under their laws against cruelty to animals.

Austria

In Austria, the Federal Act on the Protection of Animals, in Section 7, states, surgical procedures "carried out for other than therapeutic or diagnostic purposes...are prohibited, in particular...declawing."

United Kingdom

In the United Kingdom, declawing was outlawed by the Animal Welfare Act 2006, which explicitly prohibited "interference with the sensitive tissues or bone structure of the animal, otherwise than for the purposes of its medical treatment." Even before the 2006 Act, however, declawing was extremely uncommon, to the extent that most people had never seen a declawed cat. The procedure was considered cruel by almost all British vets, who refused to perform it except on medical grounds. The *Guide to Professional Conduct* of the Royal College of Veterinary Surgeons stated that declawing was "only acceptable where, in the opinion of the veterinary surgeon, injury to the animal is likely to occur during normal activity. It is not acceptable if carried out for the convenience of the owner ... the removal of claws, particularly those which are weight bearing, to preclude damage to furnishings is not acceptable."

United States

Declawing was outlawed in West Hollywood, California, in 2003, the first such ban in the US. The ordinance was authored by West Hollywood Councilmember John Duran and sponsored by The Paw Project, a non-profit organization started by Dr. Jennifer Conrad based in Santa Monica, CA. The California Veterinary Medical Association challenged the law in court. The CVMA maintained that West Hollywood had overstepped its municipal authority by enacting an ordinance that infringed on licensed professionals' state-granted rights. It did not directly address declawing as an animal welfare issue. The CVMA initially prevailed in Superior Court, but in June 2007, the California Court of Appeal overturned the lower court ruling, thus reinstating the law banning declawing in West Hollywood.

In 2004, California became the first state in the USA to enact a statewide ban on the declawing of wild and exotic cats. The bill was introduced by California Assemblymember Paul Koretz and sponsored by the Paw Project. In 2006, the United States Department of Agriculture enacted a ban on declawing of all wild and exotic animals held by USDA-licensed owners.

In April 2007, the city of Norfolk, Virginia outlawed declawing by persons other than veterinarians (Municipal Code Sec. 6.1-78.1).

In 2009, the California state legislature approved a measure, sponsored by the California Veterinary Medical Association (CVMA), intended to stop other cities from passing bans similar to West Hollywood's. The bill included all professions licensed by the state Department of Consumer Affairs, and it was signed into law by the Governor in July, 2009. However, the law's effective date, January 1, 2010, provided enough time for seven more California cities to pass local bans against the declawing of domestic cats: Los Angeles, San Francisco, Burbank, Santa Monica, Berkeley, Beverly Hills, and Culver City.

In 2012, a California bill, authored by Senator Fran Pavley and sponsored by the Paw Project, was signed into law that prohibits landlords from requiring declawing and devocalization of animals as a condition of tenancy. In 2013, the state of Rhode Island enacted a law, similar to the California law, prohibiting landlords from requiring declawing as a condition of occupancy.

Ethical Viewpoints on Declawing in the US

Declawing is widely practiced but ethically controversial within the American veterinary community. Some American and Canadian veterinarians endorse the procedure, while some have criticized and refused to perform it. Two animal protection organizations in the US, the Humane Society of the United States and the American Society for the Prevention of Cruelty to Animals, discourage the procedure. The Humane Society of the United States has supported legislation banning or restricting declawing. Multiple surveys and polls taken from 2011 reveal that the majority of United States cat owners are against declawing, believing the practice to be cruel. These surveys also suggest that the U.S. public believes that the majority of veterinarians who perform declawings only do so because of the lucrative amounts of money that can be made for performing them.

Opposition to attempts to ban or restrict declawing has come from veterinary trade organizations, such as the California Veterinary Medical Association. On the other hand, the American Veterinary Medical Association states that declawing "should be considered only after attempts have been made to prevent the cat from using its claws destructively or when its clawing presents a zoonotic risk for its owner(s)." Surveys suggest that 95% of declaw surgeries are done to protect furniture.

Alternatives to Declawing

Surgical

Tendonectomy involves cutting the deep digital flexor tendon of each claw, resulting in the cat being unable to move its distal phalanges. Without the ability to expose its claws, the cat is unable to wear down or groom its claws. For this reason, the cat subsequently requires regular nail clippings to prevent its claws from growing into its paw pads. A 1998 study published in the Journal of the American Veterinary Medical Association comparing cats undergoing onychectomy to cats undergoing tendonectomy found that, although the cats undergoing tendonectomy appeared to suffer less pain immediately post-operatively, there was no significant difference in postoperative lameness, bleeding, or infection between the two groups. A 2005 study found no evidence that tendonectomy is less painful than onychectomy. The American Veterinary Medical Association and the Canadian Veterinary Medical Association explicitly do not recommend this surgery as an alternative to declawing.

Non-surgical

According to board-certified veterinary behaviorist Dr. Gary Landsberg, "For most cats, appropriate client advice and a little effort is all that is needed to prevent scratching problems." However, many veterinary practitioners are unwilling or unable to offer solutions to behavioral problems such as scratching, other than declawing.

An effective non-surgical alternative to declawing is the application of vinyl nail caps (marketed in the US under brand names such as Soft Paws, available through veterinarians, and Soft Claws, sold through pet stores and online) that are affixed to the claws with nontoxic glue, requiring periodic replacement when the cat sheds its claw sheaths (usually every four to six weeks, depending on the cat's scratching habits).

Other alternatives include regular nail trimming; directing scratching behavior to inexpensive cardboard scratchers or scratching posts, or emery scratching pads that dull the claws; rotary sanding devices (Dremel, Pedi-Paws); covering furniture or using double-sided sticky tape or sheets such as Sticky Paws; remote aversive devices such as Scat Mats; or acceptance of cats' scratching behavior.

Docking (Dog)

Docking is the removal of portions of an animal's tail. While docking and bobbing are more commonly used to refer to removal of the tail, the term cropping is used in reference to the ears. Tail docking occurs in one of two ways. The first involves constricting the blood supply to the tail with a rubber ligature for a few days until the tail falls off. The second involves the severance of the tail with surgical scissors or a scalpel. The length to which tails are docked varies by breed, and is often specified in the breed standard.

At least 170 dog breeds have naturally occurring bob tail lines. These appear similar to docked dogs but are a distinct naturally occurring phenotype.

History

Purpose

Historically, tail docking was thought to prevent rabies, strengthen the back, increase the animal's speed, and prevent injuries when ratting, fighting, and baiting. In early Georgian times in the United Kingdom a tax was levied upon working dogs with tails, so many types of dog were docked to avoid this tax. The tax was repealed in 1796 but that did not stop the practice from persisting.

Tail docking is done in modern times either for prophylactic, therapeutic, or cosmetic purposes. For dogs that work in the field, such as some hunting dogs and herding dogs, tails can collect burrs and foxtails, causing pain and infection and, due to the tail's wagging, may be subject to abrasion or other injury while moving through dense brush or thickets.

Modern Practice

Docking of puppies younger than 10 to 14 days old is routinely carried out by both breeders and veterinarians without anesthesia. Opponents of these procedures state that most tail dockings are done for aesthetic reasons rather than health concerns and are unnecessarily painful for the dog. They point out that even non-working show or pet dogs are routinely docked. As a result, tail defects that docking proponents claim makes docking necessary in the first place are perpetuated in the breeds.They point to the many breeds of working dogs with long tails that are not traditionally docked, including English Pointers, Setters, Herding dogs, and Foxhounds.

Criticism

Robert Wansborough argued in a 1996 paper that docking tails puts dogs at a disadvantage in several ways. First, dogs use their tails to communicate with other dogs (and with people); a dog without a tail might be significantly handicapped in conveying fear, caution, aggression, playfulness, and so on.

Certain breeds use their tails as rudders when swimming, and possibly for balance when running, so active dogs with docked tails might be at a disadvantage compared to their tailed peers. In 2007, Stephen Leaver, a graduate student at the University of Victoria, published a paper on tail docking which found that tail length was important in the transmission of social cues. The study found that dogs with shorter tails (docked tails) would be approached with caution, as if the approaching dog was unsure of the emotional state of the docked dog. The study goes on to suggest that dogs with docked tails may grow up to be more aggressive. The reasoning postulated by Tom Reimchen, UVic Biologist and supervisor of the study, was that dogs who grew up without being able to efficiently transmit social cues would grow up to be more anti-social and thus more aggressive.

Wansborough also investigated seven years of records from an urban veterinary practice to demonstrate that undocked tails result in less harm than docked tails.

Influence of Kennel Clubs

Critics point out that kennel clubs with breed standards that do not make allowance for uncropped or undocked dogs put pressure on owners and breeders to continue the practice. Although the American Kennel Club (AKC) says that it has no rules that require docking or that make undocked animals ineligible for the show ring, standards for many breeds put undocked animals at a disadvantage for the conformation show ring. The American breed standard for boxers, for example, recommends that an undocked tail be "severely penalized."

The AKC position is that ear cropping and tail docking are "acceptable practices integral to defining and preserving breed character and/or enhancing good health," even though the practice is currently opposed by the American Veterinary Medical Association.

Legal Status

Today, many countries ban cropping and docking because they consider the practices unnecessary, painful, cruel or mutilation. In Europe, the cropping of ears is prohibited in all countries that have ratified the European Convention for the Protection of Pet Animals. Some countries that ratified the convention made exceptions for tail docking.

United Kingdom

Show dogs are no longer docked in the United Kingdom. A dog docked before 28 March 2007 in Wales and 6 April 2007 in England may continue to be shown at all shows in England, Wales, Scotland and Northern Ireland throughout its life. A dog docked on, or after, the above dates, regardless of where it was docked, may not be shown at shows in England and Wales where the public is charged a fee for admission. Where a working dog has been docked in England and Wales under the respective regulations, however, it may be shown where the public is charged a fee, so long as it is shown "only to demonstrate its working ability". It will thus be necessary to show working dogs in such a way as to demonstrate their working ability and not conformity to a standard. A dog legally docked in England, Wales, Northern Ireland, or abroad may be shown at any show in Scotland or Northern Ireland.

In England and Wales, ear cropping is illegal, and no dog with cropped ears can take part in any Kennel Club event (including agility and other non-conformation events). Tail docking is also illegal, except for a few working breeds; this exemption applies only when carried out by a registered veterinary surgeon.

The Royal College of Veterinary Surgeons (RCVS), the regulatory body for veterinary surgeons in the United Kingdom, has stated they consider tail docking to be "an unjustified mutilation and unethical unless done for therapeutic or acceptable prophylactic reasons". In 1995 a veterinary surgeon was brought before the RCVS disciplinary council for "disgraceful professional conduct" for carrying out cosmetic docking. The surgeon claimed that the docking was performed to prevent future injuries, and the case was dismissed for lack of evidence otherwise. Although cosmetic docking is still considered unacceptable by the RCVS, no further disciplinary action has been taken against vets performing docking.

The Animal Welfare Act 2006 makes the docking of dogs' tails a criminal offence, except for working dogs such as those used by the police force, the military, rescue services, pest control, and those used in connection with lawful animal shooting. Three options were presented to Parliament in March 2006 with Parliament opting for the second:

- An outright ban on docking dogs' tails (opposed by a majority of 278 to 267)

- A ban on docking dogs' tails with an exception for working dogs (supported by a majority of 476 to 63)

- Retention of the status quo.

Those convicted of unlawful docking are liable to a fine of up to £20,000, up to 51 weeks of imprisonment or both.

In Northern Ireland legislation known as Welfare of Animals Act (Northern Ireland) 2011 made tail docking illegal except for certain working dogs. .

In Scotland docking of any breed is illegal. The Animal Health and Welfare (Scotland) Act 2006 contains provisions prohibiting the mutilation of domesticated animals. However, the Scottish Government has carried out a consultation on this issue and have declared that they intend to legislate to bring the law in Scotland in line with the law in England and Wales, meaning that there will be an exemption for certain breeds of working dogs.

Legal Status of Dog Tail Docking and Ear Cropping by Country

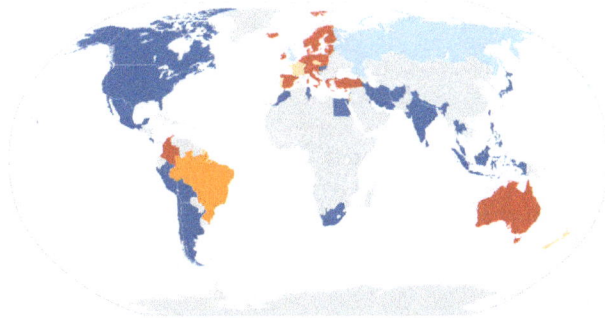

■ Unrestricted
■ Restricted (can only be performed by a vet)
■ Ear cropping banned, tail docking permitted or restricted
■ Banned for cosmetic purposes
■ Banned/Banned with few exceptions

Country	Status	Ban/restriction date (if applicable)
Afghanistan	Unrestricted	
Argentina	Unrestricted	
Australia	Banned in all states and territories.	June 2004 (East) 16 March 2010 (WA)
Austria	Banned	1 January 2005
Belgium	Banned	1 January 2006
Bolivia	Unrestricted	
Brazil	Banned for cosmetic purposes	
Bosnia and Herzegovina	Restricted: Can only be done by a vet	

| | Canada | Canada has no federal law banning pet cosmetic surgery. The Canadian Veterinary Medical Association opposes all cosmetic practices. Two provinces have provincial legislation against tail docking, ear cropping, and most cosmetic surgeries:

 • Illegal since 2015 in Prince Edward Island

 • Illegal in Newfoundland and Labrador under the Newfoundland and Labrador Regulation 35/12 on 2 May 2012.

 Three provincial veterinary associations have bans on their veterinarians performing tail docking, ear cropping, and most cosmetic surgeries:

 • Since 2008 by the New Brunswick Veterinary Medical Association (NBVMA)

 • Since 2010 by the Nova Scotia Veterinary Medical Association (NSVMA)

 • To take effect first of January 2017, a total ban on cosmetic surgery, by the Ordre des médecins vétérinaires du Québec (OMVQ)

 Three Provincial veterinary associations with ear cropping bans are open to a future ban of tail docking:

 • Since 2013 the Saskatchewan Veterinary Medical Association banned cosmetic ear cropping (bylaw 33.6)

 • Since 2015 the College of Veterinarians of British Columbia (CVBC))

 • Since 2012, Bylaw 31, by Manitoba Veterinary Medical Association (MVMA) | |

Country	Status	Date
Chile	Unrestricted	
Colombia	Banned	
Costa Rica	Unrestricted	
Croatia	Banned	
Cyprus	Banned	1991
Czech Republic	Ear cropping banned, tail docking unrestricted	
Denmark	Banned, with exceptions for five gun dog breeds	1 June 1996
Egypt	Unrestricted	
England	Ear cropping banned in 1899. Tail docking restricted since 2007, can only be done by a vet on certain working dog breeds.	2006
Estonia	Banned	2001
Finland	Banned	1 July 1996
France	Tail docking is unrestricted (France opted out of the rule regarding docking when it ratified the European Convention for the Protection of Pet Animals) Any other surgery for aesthetic purposes (such as ear cropping) is banned since 2009	
Germany	Banned, with exceptions for working gun dogs.	1 May 1998
Greece	Banned	1991
Hungary	Unrestricted	
Iceland	Banned	2001
India	Unrestricted, from Madras High Court ruling (WP № 1750/2012)	
Indonesia	Unrestricted	
Iran	Unrestricted — tail docking and ear trimming are still taught in veterinary faculties in Iran	
Ireland	Banned	7 March 2014
Israel	Banned for cosmetic purposes.	2000
Italy	Banned	
Japan	Unrestricted	
Kuwait	Unrestricted	

Country	Status	Date
Latvia	Banned	
Lebanon	Unrestricted	
Lithuania	Banned	
Luxembourg	Banned	1991
Malaysia	Unrestricted	
Morocco	Unrestricted: Morocco has no animal protection laws	
Mauritius	Unrestricted	
Mexico	Unrestricted	
Nepal	Unrestricted	
Netherlands	Banned	1 September 2001
New Zealand	Cropping ears is banned, docking tails is restricted to those trained and acting under an approved quality assurance programme in puppies less than four days old.	
Northern Ireland	Ear cropping illegal. Tail docking restricted since 2013, can only be done by a vet on certain working dog breeds.	
Norway	Banned	1987
Peru	Unrestricted	
Philippines	Unrestricted	
Portugal	Cropping ears is banned. Docking tails is allowed, as long as it's performed by a veterinarian.	2001
Poland	Banned	1997
Russia	Restricted	
Scotland	Banned	2006
Slovakia	Banned	1 January 2003
Slovenia	Banned	April 2007
South Africa	The South African Veterinary Council has banned veterinarians from performing this procedure (unless for medical purposes). Ear cropping is also banned.	1 June 2008
Spain	Banned in some autonomies	
Sri Lanka	Unrestricted	

Sweden	Banned	1989
Switzerland	Banned	1 July 1981 (ears) 1988 (tails)
Taiwan	Unrestricted	
Thailand	Unrestricted	
Tunisia	Unrestricted	
Turkey	Banned	24 June 2004
United States	Unrestricted. Some states, including New York, and Vermont have considered bills to make the practice illegal.	
Virgin Islands, British	Banned	2005
Wales	Restricted: can only be done by vet on a number of working dog breeds	2006

Cropping (Animal)

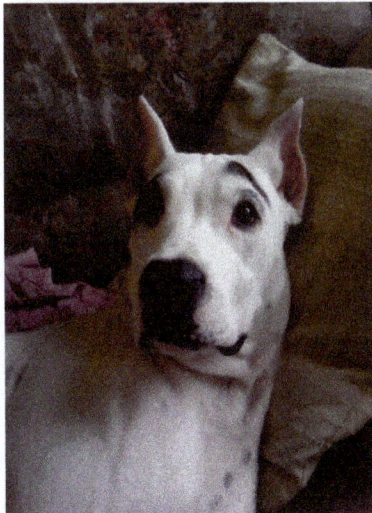

A Guatemalan Dogo with cropped ears

Cropping is the removal of part or all of the pinnae or auricles, the external visible flap of the ear, of an animal; it sometimes involves taping to make the ears pointy, Most commonly performed on dogs, it is an ancient practice that was once done for perceived health, practical or cosmetic reasons. In modern times, it is banned in many nations, but is still legal in a limited number of countries. Where permitted, it is seen only in certain breeds of dog such as the Pit bull, Doberman Pinscher, Schnauzer, Great Dane, Boxer, Caucasian Shepherd Dog and Beauceron.

The veterinary procedure is known as cosmetic otoplasty. Current veterinary science provides no medical or physical advantage to the animal from the procedure, leading to concerns over animal cruelty related to performing unnecessary surgery on the animals. In addition to the bans in place in countries around the world, it is described in some veterinary texts as "no longer considered ethical."

Cropping of large portions of the pinnae of other animals is rare, although the clipping of identifying shapes in the pinnae of livestock, called earmarks, was common prior to the introduction of compulsory ear tags. Removal of portions of the ear of laboratory mice for identification, i.e. ear-notching, is still used. The practice of cropping for cosmetic purposes is rare in non-canines, although some selectively bred animals have naturally small ears which can be mistaken for cropping.

History and Purposes

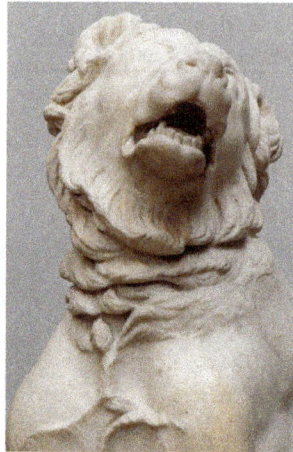

The Duncombe Dog, a 2nd-century AD Roman copy of a Hellenistic bronze, probably of the 2nd century BC and from Epirus, showing cropped ears

Ear cropping has been performed on dogs since ancient times.

Traditional Cropping

Historically, cropping was performed on working dogs in order to decrease the risk of health complications, such as ear infections or hematomas. Crops were also performed on dogs that might need to fight, either while hunting animals that might fight back or while defending livestock herds from predators, or because they were used for pit-fighting sports such as dogfighting or bear-baiting. The ears were an easy target for an opposing animal to grab or tear.

Cropping the ears of livestock guardian dogs was, and may still be, traditional in some pastoral cultures. The ears of working flock-defense dogs such as the Caucasian Shepherd Dog (Kavkazskaïa Ovtcharka) and the Pastore Maremmano-Abruzzese were traditionally cropped to reduce the possibility of wolves or aggressor dogs getting a hold on them.

According to one description, cropping was carried out when puppies were weaned, at about six weeks. It was performed by an older or expert shepherd, using the ordinary blade shears used for shearing, well sharpened. The ears were cut either to a point like those of a fox, or rounded like those of a bear. The removed auricles were given to the puppy to eat, in the belief that it would make him more "sour"; the ears were first grilled. An alternative method was to remove the ears from newborn puppies by twisting them off; however, this left almost no external ear on the dog. More than three hundred years ago, both ear-cropping and the use of spiked collars were described as a defense against wolves by Jean de la Fontaine in Fable 9 of Book X of the *Fables*, published in 1678.

Dogs may have their ears cropped, legally or not, for participation in dogfights, themselves illegal in many jurisdictions.

Health Benefits

Historically, ear cropping has been advocated as a health benefit for certain breeds with long, hanging ears. There is some evidence that dogs with standing ears may suffer from fewer ear infections than dogs with hanging ears. It has also been hypothesized that standing ears are less prone to damage and subsequent medical complications, especially in working dogs. Some claim that cropped ears enhance Boxer's hearing. Long, hanging ears can not function the same way as erect ears which can swivel toward a sound source. The erect shape directs sound waves into the ear canal and additionally amplifies the sound slightly. Long, hanging pinnae also impose a physical barrier to sound waves entering the ear canal.

Cosmetic Cropping

In the last 100 years or so, ear cropping has been performed more often for cosmetic purposes. In nations and states where it remains legal, it is usually practiced because it is required as part of a breed standard for exhibition at dog shows.

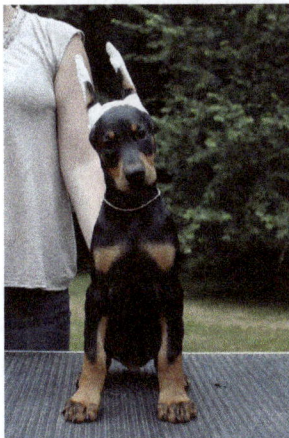

A Doberman Pinscher puppy with its ears properly taped to train them into the desired shape and carriage after cropping

The veterinary procedure is known as "cosmetic otoplasty". It is usually performed on puppies at 7 to 12 weeks of age. After 16 weeks, the procedure is more painful and the animal has greater pain memory. Up to 2/3 of the ear flap may be removed in a cropping operation, and the wound edges are closed with stitches. The ears are then bandaged and taped until they heal into the proper shape. The procedure is recommended to be undertaken under general anaesthesia; opponents primary concerns revolve around post-operative pain.

American veterinary schools do not generally teach cropping and docking, and thus veterinarians who perform the practice have to learn on the job. There are also problems with amateurs performing ear-cropping, particularly at puppy mills. Amateur cropping is not illegal in the United States, though it is highly frowned upon among prominent members of dog communities.

In the USA, although tail-docking, dewclaw removal, and neutering procedures remain common, ear-cropping is declining, save within the dog show industry. However, many show ring competitors state they would discontinue the practice altogether if they could still "win in the ring."

Animal Welfare and Law

The practice is illegal across most of Europe, including all countries that have ratified the European Convention for the Protection of Pet Animals, and most member countries of the Fédération Cynologique Internationale. It is illegal in parts of Spain and in some Canadian provinces. The situation in Italy is unclear; the ban effective 14 January 2007 may no longer be in force.

Ear-cropping is still widely practiced in the United States and parts of Canada, with approximately 130,000 puppies in the United States thought to have their ears cropped each year The American and Canadian Kennel Clubs both permit the practice. The American Kennel Club (AKC) position is that ear cropping and tail docking are "acceptable practices integral to defining and preserving breed character and/or enhancing good health." While some individual states have attempted to ban ear-cropping, there is strong opposition from some dog breed organizations, who cite health concerns and tradition.

The American Veterinary Medical Association "opposes ear cropping and tail docking of dogs when done solely for cosmetic purposes" and "encourages the elimination of ear cropping and tail docking from breed standards". Specifically, the AVMA "has recommended to the American Kennel Club and appropriate breed associations that action be taken to delete mention of cropped or trimmed ears from breed standards for dogs and to prohibit the showing of dogs with cropped or trimmed ears if such animals were born after some reasonable date". Some national chains of veterinary hospitals have voluntarily ceased to perform cosmetic surgeries on dogs. The American Humane Association opposes ear-cropping "unless it is medically necessary, as determined by a licensed veterinarian".

While it has been suggested the cropping may interfere with a dog's ability to communicate using ear signals, some also argue that cropping increases a dog's ability to communicate with ear signals. There has been no scientific comparative study of ear communication in cropped and uncropped dogs.

Status by Country

Country	Status	Ban/restriction date (if applicable)
Afghanistan	Unrestricted	
Argentina	Unrestricted	
Australia	Banned	
Austria	Banned	1 January 2005
Belgium	Banned	
Bolivia	Unrestricted	
Brazil	Banned for cosmetic purposes	
Bulgaria	Banned	2008
Canada	Canada has no federal law banning pet cosmetic surgery. The Canadian Veterinary Medical Association opposes all cosmetic alterations. Two provinces have provincial legislation prohibiting ear cropping, tail docking, and most cosmetic surgeries: Prince Edward Island (✝1) and Newfoundland and Labrador (✝2). Three province's veterinary associations ban all veterinarians from performing cosmetic surgeries on pets: New Brunswick (✝3), Nova Scotia (✝4), and Quebec (✝5) Three provincial veterinary associations have bans on ear cropping alone: Manitoba (✝6), British Columbia, and Saskatchewan (✝8).	✝1: 10 July 2015. ✝2: 1978 ✝3: 15 October 2008. ✝4: 1 April 2010. ✝5: 1 January 2017 ✝6: 3 February 2012. ✝7: 2015. ✝8: 2013
Chile	Unrestricted	
Colombia	Unclear	
Costa Rica	Unrestricted	
Croatia	Banned	
Cyprus	Banned	1993
Czech Republic	Banned	
Denmark	Banned	1 June 1996
Egypt	Unrestricted	
England	Banned	1899
Estonia	Banned	2001
Finland	Banned	1 July 1996
France	Banned, except tail-docking	1 January 2010

Germany	Banned	1 May 1992
Greece	Banned	1992
Hungary	Banned	
Iceland	Banned	2001
India	Previously restricted, currently unrestricted	
Indonesia	Unrestricted	
Ireland	Banned	
Israel	Banned	2000
Italy	Banned or unclear	
Kuwait	Unrestricted	
Latvia	Banned	
Lebanon	Unrestricted	
Lithuania	Banned	
Luxembourg	Banned	1991
Malaysia	Unrestricted	
Morocco	Unrestricted - Morocco has no animal protection laws	
Mauritius	Unrestricted	
Mexico	Unrestricted	
Nepal	Unrestricted	
Netherlands	Banned	1 September 2001
New Zealand	Banned	2004
Northern Ireland	Banned	2011
Norway	Banned	1987
Panama	Unrestricted	
Peru	Unrestricted	
Philippines	Unrestricted	
Poland	Banned	1997
Portugal	Banned	
Romania	Banned	2008
Russia	Restricted	
Scotland	Banned	1899
Slovakia	Banned	1 January 2003
Slovenia	Banned	April 2007
South Africa	Banned	June 2008
Spain	Banned in autonomies of Catalonia and Andalucia	

Sri Lanka	Unrestricted	
Sweden	Banned	1989
Switzer-land	Banned	1997
Taiwan	Unrestricted	
United States	Unrestricted (some states, including New York and Vermont, have considered bills to make the practice illegal)	2003
Virgin Is-lands	Banned	2005
Wales	Banned	1899

Naturally Small Ears

Some animals, such as the Lamancha goat, have ears which are naturally small as the result of selective breeding, and some people mistakenly believe their ears to be cropped.

In other animals, small ears may result from a genetic mutation or the emergence of a genetically recessive trait, such as in Highland cattle, where the appearance of small ears, appearing to have its pinnae cropped, is viewed as a defect.

Devocalization

Devocalization (also known as ventriculocordectomy or vocal cordectomy and when performed on dogs is commonly known as debarking or bark softening) is a surgical procedure applied to dogs and cats, where tissue is removed from the animal's vocal cords to permanently reduce the volume of their vocalizations.

Indications and Contraindications

Devocalization is usually performed at the request of an animal owner (where the procedure is legally permitted). The procedure may be forcefully requested as a result of a court order. Owners or breeders generally request the procedure because of excessive animal vocalizations, complaining neighbors, or as an alternative to euthanasia due to a court order.

Contraindications include negative reaction to anesthesia, infection, bleeding, and pain. There is also the possibility of the removed tissue growing back, or of scar tissue blocking the throat, both requiring further surgeries, though with the incisional technique, the risk of fibrosis is virtually eliminated.

Effectiveness

Canine

The devocalization procedure does not take away a dog's ability to bark. Dogs will normally bark just as much as before the procedure. After the procedure the sound will be softer, typically about half as loud as before or less, and it is not as sharp or piercing. So while the procedure does not stop barking or silence the animal completely, it is effective at reducing the sound level and sharpness of the dog's bark.

Most devocalized dogs have a subdued "husky" bark, audible up to 20 metres.

The National Council on Pet Population Study and Policy (NCPPSP) is a council of ten prominent American animal organizations which studies and addresses statistics on companion animals.

The NCPPSP's *Shelter Statistics Survey* collected data from over 5,000 shelters, The study concluded that neither excessive vocalization nor general "behavior problems" were among the top ten reasons companion animals are relinquished at shelters.

In a study of 12 shelters reporting behaviors of animals relinquished to shelters as reported by prior caretakers, a majority of relinquished cats and dogs were reported to have "rarely or never" been too noisy. Conversely, approximately 43% of dogs were reported as too noisy "sometimes", "mostly", or "always", while cats were similarly described as too noisy for approximately 26% of respondents.

Behaviors of Animals as Reported by Owners in 12 U.S. Shelters (1995–1996)				
Was too noisy	**Dogs**		**Cats**	
	Number	%	Number	%
Always	99	5.0	31	2.4
Mostly	179	9.1	67	5.2
Sometimes	575	29.2	242	18.7
Rarely/never	1,119	56.7	951	73.7

Surgical Procedure

The procedure may be performed via the animal's mouth, with a portion of the vocal folds removed using a biopsy punch, cautery tool, scissor, or laser. The procedure may also be performed via an incision in the throat and through the larynx, which is a more invasive technique. All devocalization procedures require general anesthesia.

Reasons for Excessive Vocalization

Chronic, excessive vocalization may be due to improper socialization or training, stress, boredom, fear, or frustration. Up to 35% of dog owners report problems with barking, which can cause disputes and legal problems. The practice is more common among some breeds of dog, such as the Shetland Sheepdog, which are known as loud barkers, due to the nature of the environment in which the breed was developed.

Less Invasive Interventions

Vocalizations are a natural behavior of animals which they use widely in intra-specific and inter-specific communication. As such, devocalization should generally be considered only as a last resort. Prior to this surgical intervention, there are other less invasive interventions which can be considered to overcome excessive vocalisations.

Training

Training can be one of the most effective techniques to help combat excessive barking in dogs. Acquiring the help of a professional dog trainer can often help reduce an animals barking.

Corrective Collars

The use of automatic and manual corrective collars can be useful as a training aid when used correctly; however, the use of corrective collars, particularly shock collars, is controversial and banned in some countries. Types of corrective collars include vibration, citronella spray, ultrasonic and electrostatic/shock collar.

Accommodation

Because dogs often bark excessively due to stress, boredom, or frustration, changing the aspects of an animal's environment to make them more content is a suitable way to quiet them down, rather than forcibly silencing a distressed animal. Spending more time with an animal, such as playing, walking, and other bonding activities, will keep them occupied and make them feel more at ease. If the animal is stressed, it is best to remove the object that is causing them discomfort.

Controversy and Legislation

Reasons Opposing

- In some regions of the USA and in the UK, convenience devocalization is considered a form of surgical mutilation.
- Most vets and the RSPCA offer information to behavioural schools on how to train dogs not to bark.

Reasons Favoring

- After surgery, dogs are allowed to bark more freely, which is a natural behavior.

- The dog is no longer subject to constant disapproval for its barking.

- After debarking, dogs that previously had to be kept indoors to avoid antagonizing neighbors can be allowed outdoors.

Context

Dr. Kathy Gaughan points out that "the surgery stops the barking, but it doesn't address why the dog was barking in the first place." Gaughan notes that visitors to her clinic who request debarking are usually looking for a "quick fix". Gaughan states that, commonly, those who seek debarking live in apartments, or have neighbors who complain. Gaughan also counts "breeders with many dogs" among those who most often seek convenience devocalization. However, Dr. Gaughan does not agree with those who claim the procedure is cruel, stating "Recently, some animal advocates have asserted this surgery is cruel to the animal; some countries have even outlawed the procedure. I do not believe the surgical procedure is cruel; however, failing to address the underlying factors is inappropriate."

Some breeders seek the surgery in order to limit or diminish noise levels for personal reasons ranging from convenience to prevention; some breeders even seek the surgery for puppies prior to going to new homes.

Opinions of Animal Welfare Societies

Multiple animal medicine and animal welfare organizations discourage the use of convenience devocalization, recommending that it only be used as a last resort. However, organizations such as the American Veterinary Medical Association, American Animal Hospital Association and the American Society for the Prevention of Cruelty to Animals, oppose laws that would make devocalization illegal.

The American Veterinary Medical Association's official position states that "canine devocalization should only be performed by qualified, licensed veterinarians as a final alternative after behavioral modification efforts to correct excessive vocalization have failed."

The AVMA's position was later adopted by the American Animal Hospital Association.

The Canadian Veterinary Medical Association's position statement on devocalization of dogs states: "The Canadian Veterinary Medical Association (CVMA) discourages "devocalization" of dogs unless it is the only alternative to euthanasia, and humane treatment and management methods have failed."

The American Society for the Prevention of Cruelty to Animals (ASPCA) recommends that animal caretakers first attempt to address animal behavior problems with humane behavior modification techniques and/or with a treatment protocol set up by an animal behavior specialist. The ASPCA recommends surgery only if behavior modification techniques have failed, and the animal is at risk of losing its home or its life.

Legal Restriction and Banning

The legality of convenience devocalization varies by jurisdiction.

The procedure is outlawed as a form of mutilation in the United Kingdom and all countries that have signed the European Convention for the Protection of Pet Animals. In the United States, devocalization is illegal in Massachusetts, New Jersey, and Warwick, Rhode Island.

United Kingdom

Debarking is specifically prohibited in the UK, along with ear cropping, tail docking, and declawing of cats. By law, convenience devocalization is considered a form of surgical mutilation.

United States

In the United States, laws vary by state. In 2000, anti-debarking legislation was proposed in California, New Jersey, and Ohio. The California and New Jersey bills failed, partially due to opposition from groups who predicted the ban would lead to similar bans on ear cropping and other controversial cosmetic surgical procedures on dogs. The Ohio bill survived, and was signed into law by Governor Robert Taft in August 2000. However, Ohio Revised Code 955.22 only outlawed debarking of dogs considered "vicious".

In February 2009, 15-year-old Jordan Star of Needham, Massachusetts, filed a bill to outlaw performing convenience devocalization procedures upon cats and dogs. The bill is co-sponsored by Senator Scott Brown, with the title *Logan's Law*, after a debarked sheepdog. Star said of convenience devocalization: "To take a voice away from an animal is morally wrong." The bill became state law on April 23, 2010.

Devocalizing cats and dogs became illegal in Massachusetts by state law in 2010 and in Warwick, Rhode Island, by city ordinance in 2011. Legislation to ban devocalization of dogs and cats in New York State is underway.

References

- Slatter, Douglas H. (2002) Textbook of small animal surgery 3rd edition. Philadelphia: W.B. Saunders (imprint of Elsevier Health Sciences), 2896 pages, ISBN 978-0-7216-8607-3, p.1746

- Curtis, Patricia (2002) City dog: choosing and living well with a dog in town New York: Lantern Books ISBN 978-1-59056-000-6 p.37

- Coren, Stanley (2001) How to speak dog: mastering the art of dog-human communication New

York: Simon & Schuster ISBN 978-0-7432-0297-8.

- Abraham, S. (1993). "Sad lesson learned" (PDF). American Kennel Club Gazette, American Boxer Club. Retrieved January 18, 2016.

- "Quebec's order of veterinarians bans pet cosmetic surgery". CBC News - Montreal. Canadian Broadcasting Corporation (CBC). 6 February 2016. Retrieved 20 March 2016.

- "Cosmetic ear cropping banned by B.C. veterinarians". CBC New - British Columbia. Canadian Broadcasting Corporation (CBC). 28 October 2015. Retrieved 20 March 2016.

- "European Convention for the Protection of Pet Animals". Council of Europe. Council of Europe. Retrieved 29 July 2016.

- Canadian Veterinary Medical Association. "CVMA: Devocalization of Dogs – Position Statement". Retrieved November 7, 2015.

- "Veterinary Information Network (VIN) - For Veterinarians, By Veterinarians". VIN. 2014-10-06. Retrieved 2016-05-22.

- "Cropping and Docking: A Discussion of the Controversy and the Role of Law in Preventing Unnecessary Cosmetic Surgery on Dogs". Animallaw.info. Retrieved 2013-04-17.

- "Tail docking illegal in Australia". RSPCA Australia. 3 August 2010. Archived from the original on 13 December 2007. Retrieved 2012-01-18.

- "Ear cropping of dogs banned in Manitoba". CBC News - Manitoba. Canadian Broadcasting Corporation (CBC). 10 February 2012. Retrieved 19 March 2016.

Veterinary Medicine: Tools and Equipments

An Elizabethan collar is a medical device that is worn by animals; it is shaped like a cone and its main purpose is to prevent the animal from biting its own body. This is done so that the wound that the animal has is properly healed. Dog crate, nose ring, livestock crush, screw picket, muzzle and elastration are some of the tools and equipments used in veterinary medicine. The aspects elucidated in this chapter are of vital importance, and provide a better understanding of veterinary medicine.

Elizabethan Collar

An Elizabethan collar, E-Collar, or pet cone, (sometimes humorously called a pet lampshade, pet radar dish or cone of shame) is a protective medical device worn by an animal, usually a cat or dog. Shaped like a truncated cone, its purpose is to prevent the animal from biting or licking at its body or scratching at its head or neck while wounds or injuries heal.

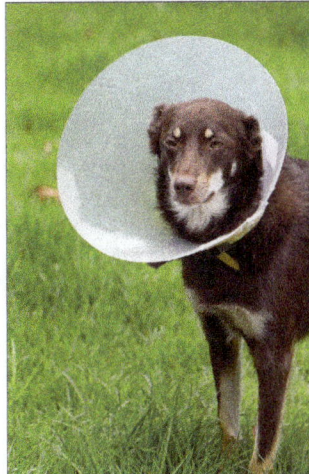

An Australian Kelpie wearing an Elizabethan collar in order to help an eye infection to heal.

The device is generally attached to the pet's usual collar with strings or tabs passed through holes punched in the sides of the plastic. The neck of the collar should be short enough to let the animal eat and drink. Although most pets adjust to them quite well, others will not eat or drink with the collar in place and the collar is temporarily removed for meals.

While purpose-made collars can be purchased from veterinarians or pet stores, they can also be made from plastic and cardboard or by using plastic flowerpots, wastebaskets, buckets or lampshades. Modern collars might involve soft fabric trim along the edges to increase comfort and velcro surfaces for ease of attachment and removal.

The collars are named from the ruffs worn in Elizabethan times. They were invented in the early 1960's by Frank L. Johnson.

Types of Collars

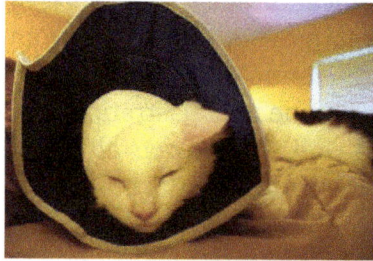

A soft fabric collar

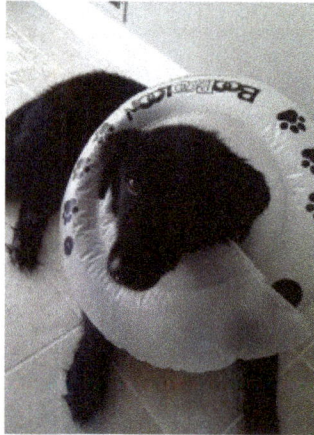

An inflatable Elizabethan collar. These collars are designed to be more comfortable and allow pets easier access to food and water.

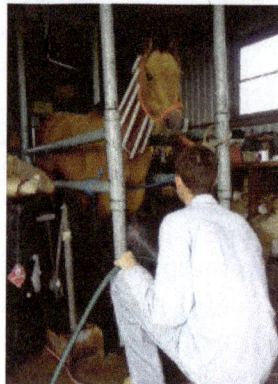

Horse "neck cradle"

Dog Crate

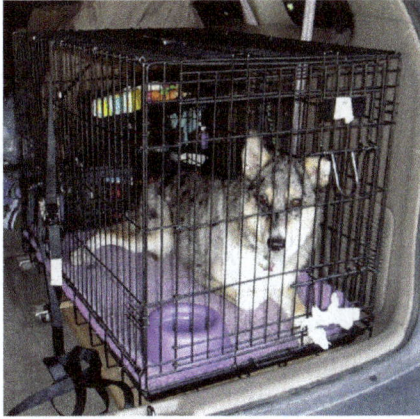

One variety of wire crate

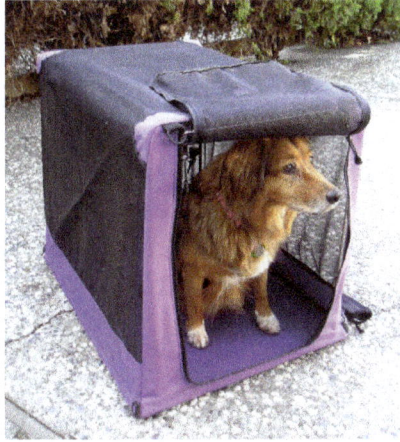

A variety of a soft crate

A dog crate is a metal, wire, plastic, or fabric enclosure with a door in which a dog may be kept for security or transportation. Dog crates are designed to replicate a dog's natural den and as such can provide them with a place of refuge at home or when traveling to new surroundings. Crate training accustoms the dog with the crate. The most common reasons for using a dog crate are for toilet training a new puppy, taking a dog on short trips inside the car, displaying them at a dog show, or giving a dog a place to go when visitors come to the house. Similarly as people can have their own room to "enjoy a moment of solace, your dog likes having its own room … a little, cozy place of their own … dog crates offer a superlative home for your dog where it can feel safe and secure." Using a crate for a dog is similar to having a playpen for a toddler or a crib for a baby, and allows the owner to take their eyes off their pet. Additionally, covering a crate with a blanket, putting your pet's favorite toys inside, and having enough packaging inside the cage to ensure your pet does not get hurt in the move are all things that will improve a pet's move.

Types of Dog Crates

There are many types of dog crates, and variations within the types. The factors to consider include cost, durability, portability, and style.

- Solid plastic crates are usually more suitable than other types for secure travel, such as in an airplane. They might also be safer in a car accident than other types. Disadvantages are that they take up a lot of space and do not fold for storage.

- Crash tested steel crates are designed specifically for use in hatchbacks and SUVs for pet vehicle transportation. They have special crumple zones designed to work with the crumple zones of the vehicles and absorb the impact of the accident and have been lab tested for safety. These crates are not intended for use on airplanes or for carrying pets outside of vehicles. They also do not make good housebreaking crates.

- Aluminum crates can be either fixed or folding. A few of their advantages are: light weight, very strong when constructed with appropriate bracing, will not rust, excellent airflow and vision for the dogs. Aluminum crates are suitable for use at veterinary hospitals, car travel, as a permanent "den" for your dog inside the home and in breeding kennel environments. Some aluminum crates have solid walls and some have bars. The crates with bars may be more suitable for dogs who need to see out to feel comfortable. Other dogs may prefer the den like feel of the solid wall variety to feel secure.

- Wire crates usually can be folded for storage or transport, although it might be difficult to do and they are fairly heavy for their size. They provide more airflow for the dog and provide people with a clearer view inside and they range in size. Such crates are often used in car travel, at veterinary hospitals, and at kennels. There are a variety of covers and pads available to make crates safe and more comfortable.

  Wire crates are also popular at dog shows; they allow the dog to be clearly seen by spectators, and sashes, rosettes, and ribbons won can be hung on the crate for display.

- Soft crates can be easily folded for storage or transport and are lightweight. They provide the dog with a stronger sense of security but still allow visibility and airflow. They cannot be used with dogs who are likely to dig or chew at the crate, and they are unsuitable for transporting dogs in vehicles.

- Dog tents are an alternative to soft crates. They offer many of the same advantages (and disadvantages) of soft crates but fold down to an even smaller size and are ultra lightweight so that they can be stuffed into tent bags and taken virtually anywhere. They are good enclosures for dog owners who need to pack their soft crates into cramped vehicles or suitcases or for people who hike, camp, or are involved in dog sports. Like soft crates, they are not suitable for dogs who are not housebroken, or for vehicle travel.

Nose Ring (Animal)

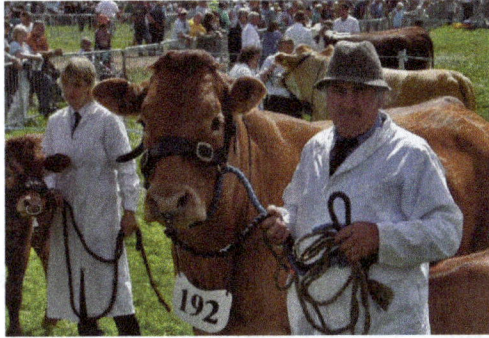

Show halters and bulldog nose rings on cattle at an agricultural show in the United Kingdom

A nose ring is a ring made of metal designed to be installed through the nasal septum of domestic cattle, usually bulls. Nose rings are often required for bulls when exhibited at agricultural shows. There also is a clip-on ring design used for controlling other cattle for showing or handling. Nose rings are also used to prevent pigs rooting, and to encourage the weaning of young calves and other livestock by discouraging them from suckling.

History

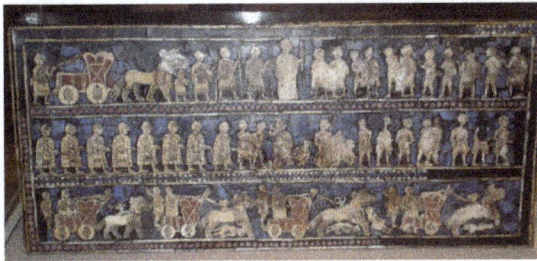

The Standard of Ur

Historically, the use of nose rings for controlling animals dates to the dawn of recorded civilization. They were used in ancient Sumer and are seen on the Standard of Ur, where they were used on both draught cattle and equines.

Use

The nose ring assists the handler to control a dangerous animal with minimal risk of injury or disruption by exerting stress on one of the most sensitive parts of the animal, the nose. Bulls, especially, are powerful and sometimes unpredictable animals which, if uncontrolled, can kill or severely injure a human handler.

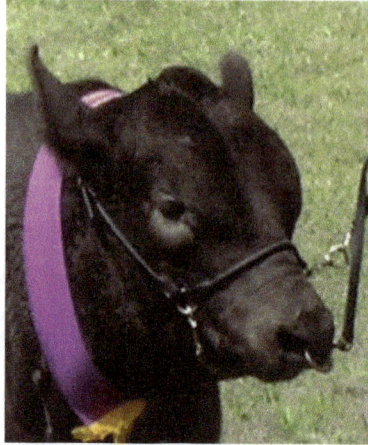

A nose ring is used to maintain control of this bull being exhibited at a livestock show.

Control of the bull may be done by holding the ring by hand, looping a piece of rope through it, clipping on a lead rope, or clipping on a stiff *bull pole* (*bull staff*). A rope or chain from the ring may be attached to a bull's horns or to a head-collar for additional control.

With an aggressive bull, a short length of chain or rope may be left hanging loose from the ring, so when he ducks in a threatening manner, the bull will step on the chain and be deterred from attacking. This lead may also facilitate capture and control of a frisky bull.

Construction and Insertion

Bull rings are usually about 3 to 5 inches (8 to 13 cm) in diameter, depending on the size of the bull. Bull rings are commonly made from aluminium, stainless steel or copper, in the form of a pair of hinged semicircles, held closed by a small brass bolt whose head is broken off during installation. If a ring needs to be removed (for example, if the bull has grown out of it), it is cut or unscrewed.

The ring is normally placed on the bull between 9 and 12 months of age. It is usually done by a veterinarian, who pierces the septum with a scalpel or punch. Self-piercing rings (with sharp ends designed to be pressed through the septum and then pulled together with a screw) have been available for many years; these are also usually installed by a veterinarian rather than the farmer.

Other Designs

Calf-weaning Ring

Calf-weaning nose rings or nosebands provide an alternative to separating calves from their mothers during the weaning period. They have plastic spikes which are uncomfortable for the cow, causing her to reject the calf's efforts at suckling. Weaning nose rings are also available for sheep and goats. These nose rings (usually made of plastic) clip onto the nose without piercing it, and are reusable.

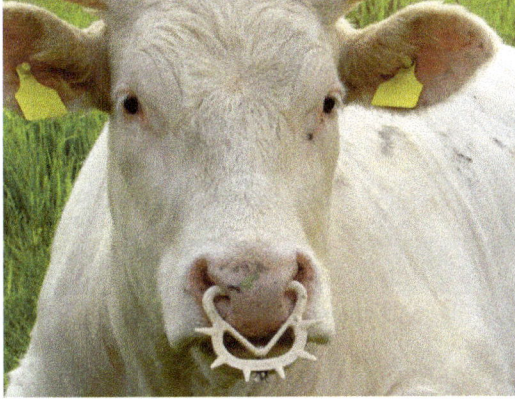

A spiked ring which prevents suckling

Bulldogs

Self-locking or spring-closing show-lead nose rings, also called "bulldogs" or nose grips, are removable rings that do not require the nose to be pierced. They are often used on steers and cows, along with a halter, at agricultural shows, or when handling cattle for examination, marking or treatment. They stay shut until released, and usually have a loop for the attachment of a cord or lead rope. They give similar control to a bull ring without the need for permanent attachment.

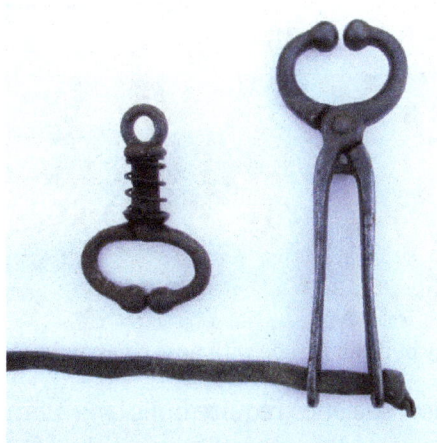

Show-lead nose ring (bulldogs), and bull tongs or bull-holders on the right

Bull Tongs

Bull-holders, also known as bull-tongs, have a pliers action and are used for short periods on grown cattle when they are being mouthed or drenched. A chain, rope or strap keeps the grips closed and may be passed over a bar at the front of a head bail to elevate the head. The thumb and forefinger may also used in this way on smaller animals.

Pig Rings

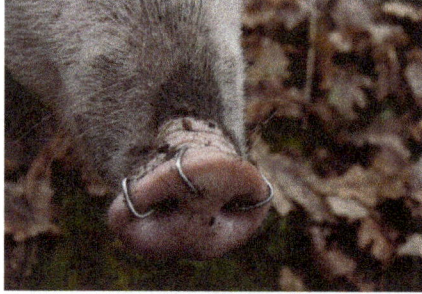

Nose rings on a young pig foraging on the New Forest

Pigs dig or "root" with their snouts, and such digging may be undesirable in some circumstances. Nose rings make digging uncomfortable for the animal, although a rung pig is still able to forage freely through leaf litter and surface vegetation. Pig ringing may sometimes be required by local regulations, as when pigs are turned out for pannage in public woods (such as on the New Forest in southern England).

Pig rings usually consist of open copper or steel wire rings with sharp ends, about one inch (about 2.5 cm) in diameter. These are clipped to the rim of the nose, not through the nostrils. Typically an adult pig will be given three or four rings, as they may sometimes become dislodged. Alternatively a ring may be placed through the septum, similarly to a bull's ring.

Bull Handling in the Show Ring

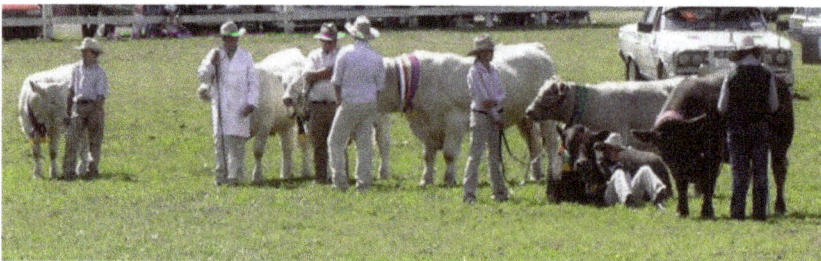

Charolais & Murray Grey bulls on parade with nose rings and a show lead ring, Australia

For safety reasons, many show societies require bulls over 12 months to be led with a nose ring. A bull may be led by a rope tied through the ring, although a halter (headcollar) is usually also used so as not to rely unduly on the nose ring for control. If the bull has horns, the lead rope may also be fastened around those and then passed down through the nose ring. Some shows require other cattle to be led with nose grips (bulldogs). Several methods exist for handling a bull with a ring installed. One method of leading a bull is to have one person on either side of the bull with both halter lead ropes through the ring, which prevents the bull from gaining pace and also from running into the handlers. Another practice is for one handler to use a rope and the other a bull-staff attached to the ring.

Bull Handling on the Farm or Ranch

It is estimated that 42% of all livestock-related human fatalities are a result of bull attacks, and only about one in twenty victims of a bull attack survives. Dairy breed bulls are particularly dangerous and unpredictable; the hazards of bull handling are a significant cause of injury and death for dairy farmers in some parts of the United States. Most cattle breeders recognize the importance of looking after expensive bulls that are expected to improve herds and profits. Nonetheless, the dangers of bull handling, particularly from dairy bulls in close quarters, are regularly proven by the obituaries. Good bull management and safety practices require caution in handling beef and dairy bulls, and use of the nose ring and chain is a recommended precaution for modern farmers.

However, in many regions, particularly in the beef industry, bulls do not have nose rings unless they are to be exhibited and they are generally driven about as other cattle would be. Cows with young calves can be particularly dangerous if protecting their young, and cattle in general, including calves, steers and bullocks, do cause many serious human injuries and deaths.

Generally the use of both a ring and a halter, and management of the bull by two people, is the preferred method today for controlling the bull. Typically, a bull was led by a wooden staff with a steel end that snapped into the ring. A long rigid steel or wooden bull staff locked into the ring could also be used to push a bull out of a pen without requiring the handler to enter the pen for cleaning or feeding. Because of the risk that the bull may drive the staff into the handler if the bull misbehaves many handlers prefer to avoid their use nowadays. One current veterinary text still recommends the use of a staff in addition to the halter:

Many handlers rely on a nose ring to control a bull. But a ring in his nose is no good unless you have a bull staff and use it. A bull staff is a pole with a snap in the end that clips to the bull ring. Leading a bull with a staff gives you a lot more handling power as the bull can't get any closer to you than the length of the staff allows. Leading him only by a chain in the ring lets him run over you at will.

Most dairy or beef farms traditionally had at least one, if not several, bulls for breeding purposes. The handling of an aggressive, powerful animal was a practical issue with life-threatening consequences for the farmer. The need to move the bull in and out of its pen to cover cows exposed the farmer to serious jeopardy of life and limb. Being trampled, jammed against a wall or gored by a bull was one of the most frequent causes of death in the dairy industry prior to 1940. As suggested in one popular farming magazine, "Handle [the bull] with a staff and take no chances. The gentle bull, not the vicious one, most often kills or maims his keeper."

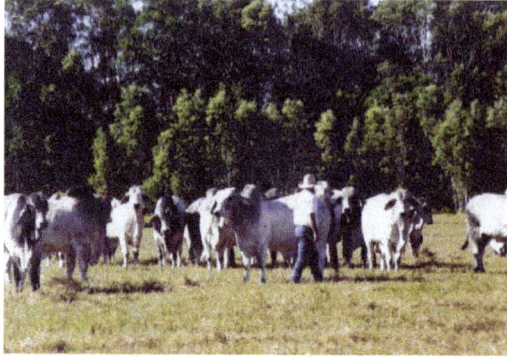

Bulls respond well to a good handler

When allowed outside its pen, the bull typically was kept in a halter connected by a strap snapped into the ring in his nose for ease of control. In the bull pen, the use of a ring connected by a cable to a fixed point was recommended as a means of controlling and securing the bull while allowing a degree of movement by the subject bull. If the pen was strong enough, the bull could be turned loose, and if needed, placed in a stanchion. Farmers who lacked an assistant, or a bull staff, had no choice but to adopt other means. Some farmers elected to move their bulls by tying a rope to the ring and tying the other end of the rope to a farm tractor, providing both motive power and a degree of protection from the angry bull. The efficacy of this technique is doubtful, and may depend on the size of the tractor and of the bull; one authority has "seen a bull lift the front end of a tractor like a toy". Others used dogs and horses. Not all farmers could afford specially designed and manufactured bull handling products, which were not readily available until the 1980s. The experimental improvisation of techniques for bull handling, as in many aspects of family farming, was a common practice.

Livestock Crush

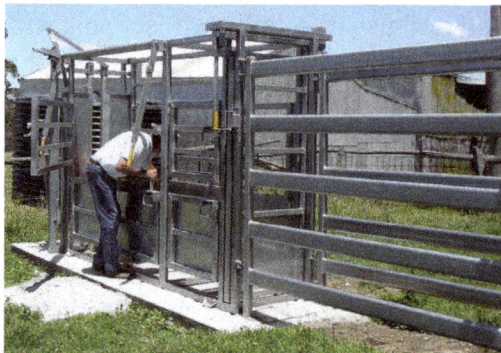

A cattle crush and an anti-bruise race in Australia.

A cattle crush (in UK, New Zealand, Ireland and Australia), squeeze chute (North America), standing stock, or simply stock (North America, Ireland) is a strongly built stall or cage for holding cattle, horses, or other livestock safely while they are examined, marked, or given veterinary treatment. Cows may be made to suckle calves in a crush. For the safety of the animal and the people attending it, a close-fitting crush may be used to ensure the animal stands "stock still". The overall purpose of a crush is to hold an animal still to minimise the risk of injury to both the animal and the operator while work on the animal is performed.

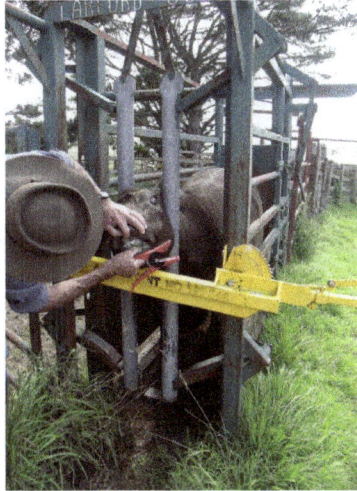

Chin (or neck) bar in operation during mouthing.

Construction

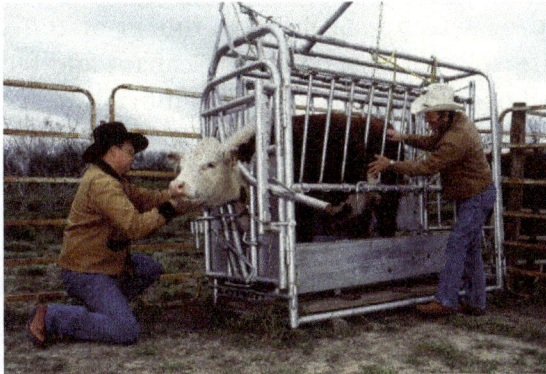

A portable crush

Crushes were traditionally manufactured from wood; this, however, was prone to deterioration from the elements over time, as well as having the potential to splinter and cause injury to the animal. In recent years, most budget-quality crushes have been built using standard heavy steel pipe that is welded together, while superior quality crushes are now manufactured using doubly symmetric oval tubing for increasing bending strength, bruise minimisation and stiffness in stockyard applications. In Australia, the steel itself should ideally be manufactured to High Tensile Grade 350LO - 450LO and conform to Australian Standards AS 1163 for structural steel.

Cattle crushes may be fully fixed or mobile; however, most crushes are best classified as semipermanent, being potentially movable but designed to primarily stay in one place. A cattle crush is typically linked to a *cattle race* (also known as an *alley*). The front end has a *head bail* (or *neck yoke* or *head gate*) to catch the animal and may have a baulk gate that swings aside to assist in catching the beast. The bail is often adjustable to accommodate animals of different sizes. This bail may incorporate a chin or neck bar to hold the animal's head still. A side lever operates the head bail to capture the animals, with the better types having a rear drop-away safety lever for easier movement of the cattle into the bail. Usually, smaller animals can walk through the head bails incorporated in crushes.

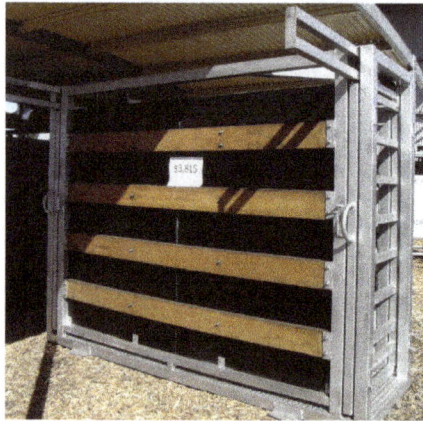

Scanning and weighing crush with timber and belting sides to increase the accuracy of ear tag scanning.

Lower side panels and/or gates of sheet metal, timber or conveyor belting are used in some cases to ensure animals' legs do not get caught and reduce the likelihood of operator injury. At least one side gate is usually split to allow access to various parts of the animal being held, as well as providing access to feed a calf, amongst other things. A *squeeze crush* has a manual or hydraulic mechanism to squeeze the animal from the sides, immobilizing the animal while keeping bruising to a minimum. A sliding entrance gate, operated from the side of the crush, is set a few feet behind the captured animal to allow for clearance and prevent other animals entering. Crushes will, in many cases, have a single or split veterinary gate that swings behind the animal to improve operator safety, while preventing the animal from moving backwards by a horizontal *rump bar* inserted just behind its haunches into one of a series of slots. If this arrangement is absent, a palpation cage can be added to the crush for veterinary use when artificial insemination or pregnancy testing is being performed, or for other uses. Older crushes can also be found to have a guillotine gate that is also operated from the side via rope or chain where the gate is raised up for the animal to go under upon entering the crush, and then let down behind the animal.

A crush is a permanent fixture in slaughterhouses, because the animal is carried on a conveyor restrainer under its belly, with its legs dangling in a slot on either side. Carried in this manner, the animal is unable to move either forward or backward by its own volition.

Some mobile crushes are equipped with a set of wheels so they can be towed from yard to yard. A few of these portable crushes are built so the crush may also be used as a portable loading ramp. A mobile crush must incorporate a strong floor, to prevent the animal moving it by walking along the ground.

Crushes vary in sophistication, according to requirements and cost. The simplest are just a part of a cattle race (alley) with a suitable head bail. More complex ones incorporate features such as automatic catching systems, hatches (to gain access to various parts of the animal), winches (to raise the feet or the whole animal), constricting sides to hold the animal firmly (normal in North American slaughterhouses), a rocking floor to prevent kicking or a weighing mechanism.

Specialist Crushes

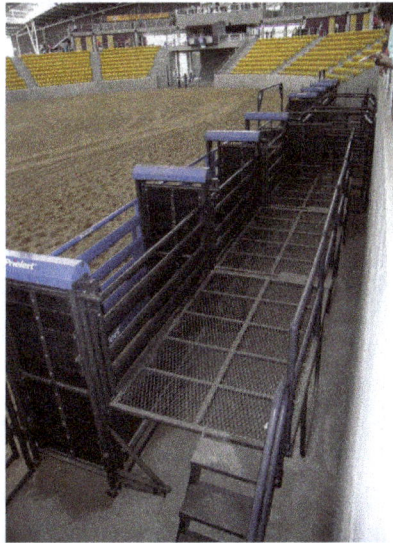

Indoor rough-riding chutes, AELEC, Tamworth, New South Wales.

Specialist crushes are made for various purposes. For example, those designed for cattle with very long horns (such as Highland cattle or Texas Longhorn cattle) are low-sided or very wide, to avoid damage to the horns. Other specialist crushes include those for tasks such as automatic scanning, foot-trimming or clipping the hair under the belly, and smaller crushes (calf cradles) for calves.

Standing stocks for cattle and horses are more commonly stand-alone units, not connected to races (alleys) except for handling animals not accustomed to being handled. These stand-alone units may be permanent or portable. Some portable units disassemble for transport to shows and sales. These units are used during grooming and also with veterinary procedures performed with the animal standing, especially if it requires heavy sedation, or to permit surgery under sedation rather than general anesthesia. For some surgical procedures, this is reported to be efficient. These units also are used during some procedures that require a horse to stand still, but without sedation.

There are two different types of specialised crushes used in rodeo arenas. Those for the "rough stock" events, such as bronc riding and bull riding, are known as bucking chutes or rough-riding chutes. For events such as steer roping, the crush is called a roping chute. The rough-riding chutes are notably higher in order to hold horses and adult bulls, and have platforms and rail spacing that allows riders and assistants to access the animal from above. These chutes release the animal and the rider through a side gate. A roping chute is large enough to contain a steer of the size used in steer wrestling and may have a seat above the chute for an operator. The steer or calf is released through the front of the chute.

Hoof Trimming Crush

A hoof trimming crush, also called a hoof trimming chute or hoof trimming stalls, is a crush specifically designed for the task of caring for cattle hooves, specifically trimming excess hoof material and cleaning. Such crushes range from simple standing frameworks to highly complex fixed or portable devices where much or all of the process is mechanised. Many standard crushes now come with optional fitting kits to add to a non foot trimming crush.

Integrated Weighing Systems

In recent years, Crushes are often integrated with weighing systems. The crush provides the ideal opportunity to weigh and measure the animal while it is safely contained within the unit.

History

Many cattle producers managed herds with nothing more than a race (alley) and a headgate (or a rope) until tagging requirements and disease control necessitated the installation of crushes.

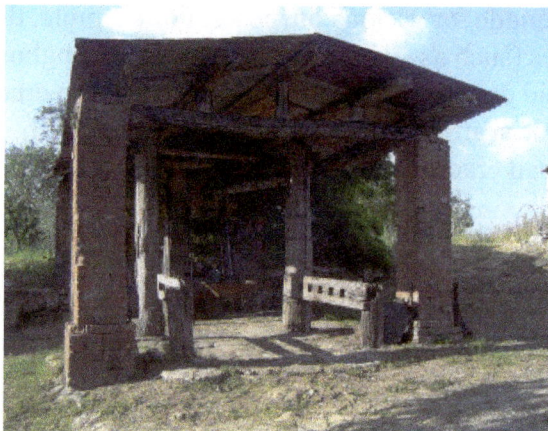

Roofed ox shoeing crush of three-column construction in Pievasciata, Castelnuovo Berardenga, Siena, Italy

In the past the principal use of the crush, in England also known as a trevis, was for the shoeing of oxen. Crushes were, and in places still are, used for this purpose in North America and in many European countries. They were usually stand-alone constructions of heavy timbers or stone columns and beams. Some were simple, without a head bail or yoke, while others had more sophisticated restraints and mechanisms; a common feature is a belly sling which allows the animal to be partly or wholly raised from the ground. In Spain, the crush was a village community resource and is called *potro de herrar*, or "shoeing frame". In France it is called *travail à ferrer* (plural *travails*, not *travaux*) or "shoeing trevis", and was associated with blacksmith shops. In central Italy it is called a *travaglio*, but in Sardinia is referred to as Sardinian: *sa macchina po ferrai is boisi*, or "the machine for shoeing the oxen". In the United States it was called an ox sling, an ox press or shoeing stalls. In some countries, including the Netherlands and France, horses were commonly shod in the same structures. In the United States similar but smaller structures, usually called horse shoeing stocks, are still in use, primarily to assist farriers in supporting the weight of the horse's hoof and leg when shoeing draft horses.

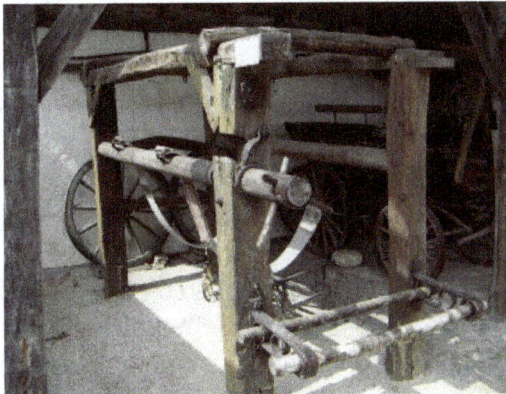

Ox shoeing sling in the Dorfmuseum of Mönchhof, Austria; a pair of ox shoes is attached to the near left column

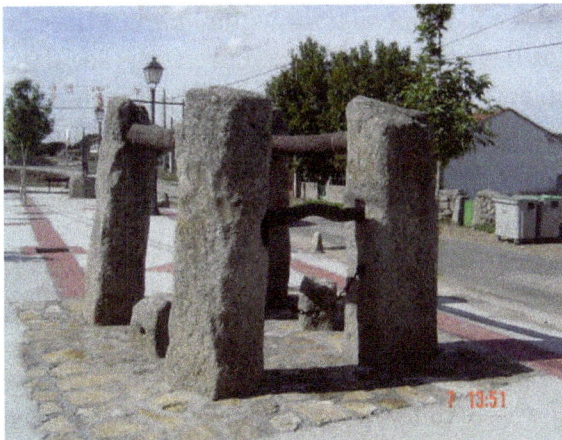

In Villar de Corneja (Ávila), Spain, the community *potro de herrar* includes a piece of the yoke used to limit movement of the animal's head.

Hartmann Alligator Forceps

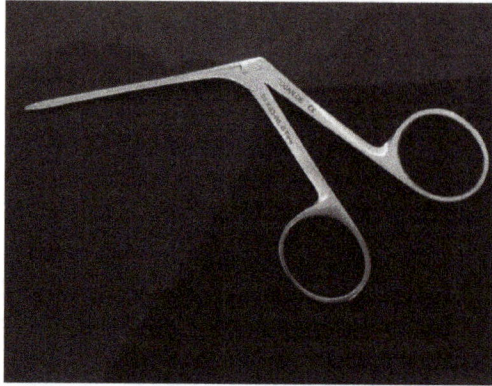

Hartmann Alligator Forceps, 8 cm / 3,14 inch, fine

The Hartmann alligator forceps or Hartmann foreign body forceps are named after the German physician Arthur Hartmann medical forceps for removing foreign bodies. It is used in addition to surgery mainly in Otorhinolaryngology (ENT). More than 80% of the Hartmann alligator forceps are produced in Pakistan in small workshops handmade in many variations of the mouth. Their quality depends on the origin and quality of the stainless steel. Indian steel is used often for hobbyist use. FDA and CE certified instruments also veterinary instruments are normal made in Japanese or German steel. The shaft length varies up to one meter, is predominantly 8 to 12 cm. Only the top mouth opens alligator-like. (in US therefore has the medical term "Alligator Mouth" or "Hartmann Alligator Forceps" enforced. A common name also is "Crocodile forceps"). The standard length of the muzzle from the front hinge implementation is 1.5 cm or 1 cm. Thus, the clamp is used where normal tweezers or fine instruments are struggling to grasp small objects. So you can even grasp objects in small tubes and position them precisely.

The ear clamp is used wherever exist problems with normal tweezers or fine instruments to grasp small objects. It opens only a small part of the mouth. So you can even grasp objects in small tubes and position them precisely. Ideal during soldering, when it is difficult to position accurately small components. In veterinary medicine the Hartmann, Ear Polypus Forcep is used to remove awns or epilate hairs of dogs ears. The design reduces the natural tremor (shaking).

Screw Picket

A screw picket is a metal device which is used to secure objects to the ground. Today, screw pickets are used widely to temporarily "picket" dogs. They are also used to graze animals such as sheep, goats, and horses. Screw pickets are also used to stabilize small trees, tent poles, and other objects that are intended to remain upright.

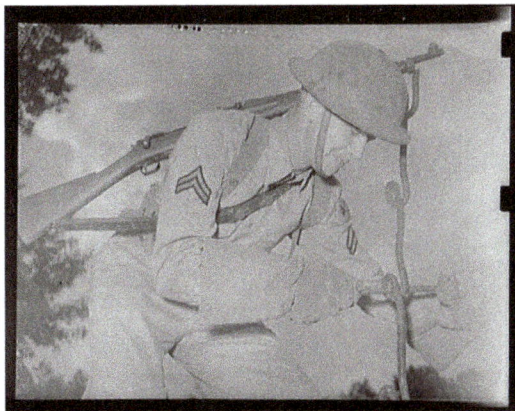

A soldier using a barbed wire anchor spike to screw in a picket at Fort Belvoir, Virginia (August, 1942)

The original picket was a stake hammered into the ground to secure a horse by tying it to the stake. This required a second tool (a hammer) or the availability of a rock to use instead of a tool. The screw picket is screwed (by turning it) into the ground. In hard ground, it requires a second tool (a leverage bar, or a spare screw picket) or the availability of a length of wood. Screw pickets can be easily bent or broken, but less easily pulled from the ground.

Military Non-equestrian use

Screw pickets (used as supports for barbed wire defences) were introduced c. 1915 as a replacement for timber posts. The French name for this type of "steel stake" was "queue de cochon" or pigtail. The World War I steel stake became known in the British Army as a "corkscrew picket". The corkscrew picket was made from a steel bar which had its bottom end bent into a spiral coil. It also had three loops or "eyes" (some even had four) formed, one at top, one at midway and one just above the corkscrew spiral. The final product was about eight feet long.

Groups of soldiers known as wiring parties went out at night into no man's land to position these supports. They later strung the barbed wire through the loops to form a defensive wire obstacle as a protection for their trench line. The British called this type of stake a 'corkscrew' picket because it was screwed into the ground rather than hammered in as the timber posts had been (the hammering made loud noise, usually attracting enemy fire). The screw pickets replaced the timber posts (although screw pickets were less rigid than timber posts), because they could be installed rapidly and silently. A wiring party is described in detail in World War I novel *All Quiet on the Western Front* by contemporary author Erich Maria Remarque.

The corkscrew picket was screwed into the ground by turning it in a clockwise direction using an entrenching tool's handle or a stick inserted in the bottom eye of the picket for leverage. The bottom eye was used in order to avoid bending the vertical bar of the picket.

Muzzle (Device)

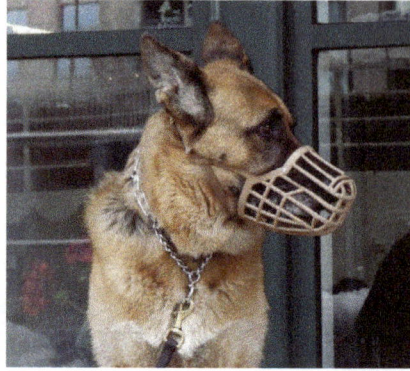

A muzzled German Shepherd

A muzzle is a device that is placed over the snout of an animal to keep it from biting or otherwise opening its mouth.

Muzzles can be primarily solid, with air holes to allow the animal to breathe, or formed from a set of straps that provides better air circulation and allow the animal to drink, and in some cases, eat. Leather, wire, plastic, and nylon are common materials for muzzles. The shape and construction of the muzzle might differ depending on whether the intent is to prevent an animal from biting or from eating, for example.

Dog Muzzles

Muzzles are sometimes used on untrained dogs, large or small, to prevent unwanted biting or scavenging. They can also be used on dogs who display aggression, whether motivated by excitement, fear or prey drive. They are usually made with a strong buckle or other fastening device to ensure that they do not come off accidentally. Muzzles are also used on dogs when there is a risk of them taking baits that have been laid for vermin. The most suitable materials for dog muzzles are leather, nylon, plastic and others. The most comfortable muzzles for dogs are those with wire cage construction. Muzzles of this kind give enough freedom for a dog to eat, drink and freely pant. The latter two are of vital importance, especially in hot weather.

Dog muzzles can be found in most pet supply stores.

Equine Muzzles

Certain muzzles with a wire-like structure are used on horses and related animals, usually to prevent biting or cribbing. Other types, known as "grazing muzzles", have a small opening in the center that allows limited intake of grass, and are used on obese horses or on those animals prone to laminitis or choke, to prevent them from eating too much or too fast.

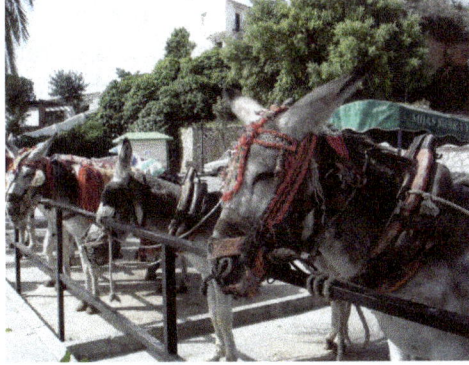

Donkeys wearing muzzles

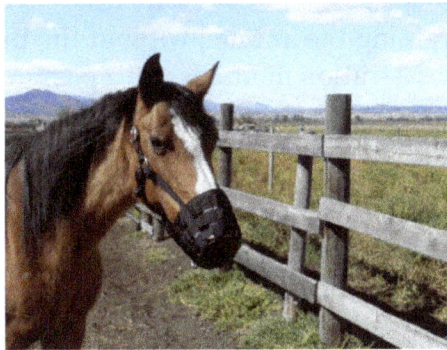

A grazing muzzle on a horse

Horses trained for airscenting, for search and rescue or police work, often are worked in muzzles. This helps to keep them focused on their work, because they cannot easily snatch bites of grass.

Horse muzzles may be purchased in tack shops or from equestrian supply companies, and are available as a halter attachment, or as a separate piece of equipment.

Elastration

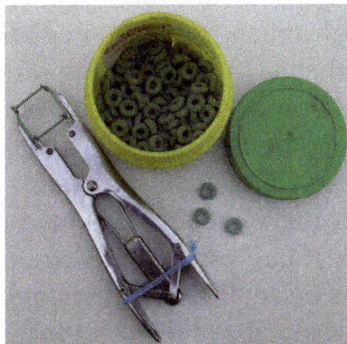

Rubber elastrator rings and pliers

Elastration (a portmanteau of "elastic" and "castration") is a bloodless method of male castration and docking commonly used for livestock. Elastration is simply banding the body part (scrotum or tail) until it drops off. This method is favored for its simplicity, low cost, and minimal training requirements.

Castration

Elastration is the most common method used to castrate sheep and goats, but is also common in cattle.

Procedure

Elastration involves restraining the animal, without the need for anesthesia or sedation (unlike most other castration methods), in a position that provides access to the genitals. Special *elastrator pliers* are then used to place a tight latex (rubber) *elastrator ring* gently around the base of the scrotum. This cuts the blood supply to the scrotum and testicles, which will totally decay and slough off within a few weeks. Care must be taken during the procedure to ensure that both testicles are fully descended and properly located inside the scrotum, and that the animal's nipples are not included within the ring. Elastration is normally limited to castrations done during the first few weeks of life, and it cannot be used for species where the scrotum does not have a narrow base, such as pigs or horses. It is commonly recommended to not use this method on goats until they are 4–6 weeks in ages. This is due to possible complications that could occur later in life. There are those who feel that this method is inhumane and choose to use other methods. These methods would include what some call the "Emasculatome", "Burdizzo",or "Richey Nipper". The Burdizzo and Richey Nipper are names of tools used for the process of the emasculatome.

Possible Complications

Some European countries have banned the practice due to their belief that the procedure is inhumane. There is some evidence that elastration is more painful if carried out on older animals, although much of the immediate pain of application can be prevented by injection of local anaesthesia into the scrotal neck and testicles. Practitioners usually try to elastrate as soon as possible, once the testicles have descended, to reduce the amount of dead tissue, infection, and accompanying complications. However, with some animals such as goats, castrating too early increases the frequency of kidney stones and urinary problems due to reduced size of the urethra, so elastration may be postponed. If bull calves are castrated within the first one or two days the testes may sometimes be small and soft enough to be drawn up through the ring, and they continue to develop above the scrotum – surgical castration then becomes necessary.

Docking

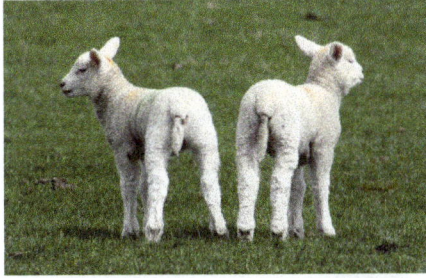

Lambs with rubber rings on their tails

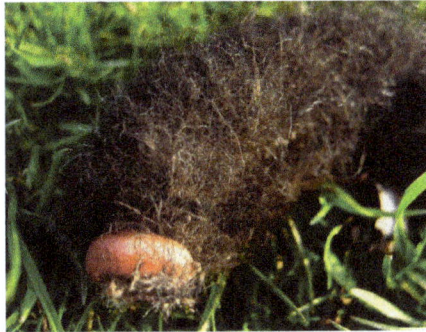

Elastrated lamb tail

The same tool and rings are also used to dock the tails of many breeds of sheep, to pre-vent dung building up on the tails (which can lead to fly strike). This is usually done at the same time as castration of the ram lambs. Its also called sheep marking in Australia.

Halter

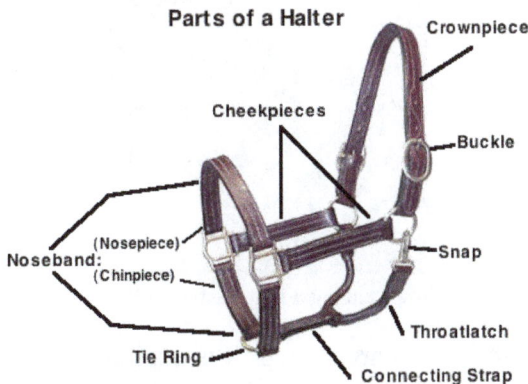

Parts of a Halter

A leather "Newmarket headcollar" (UK) or "stable halter" (US) for horses

A halter (US) or headcollar (UK) is headgear that is used to lead or tie up livestock and, occasionally, other animals; it fits behind the ears (behind the poll), and around the muzzle. To handle the animal, usually a lead rope or lead shank is attached. On smaller animals, such as dogs, a leash is attached to the halter.

History

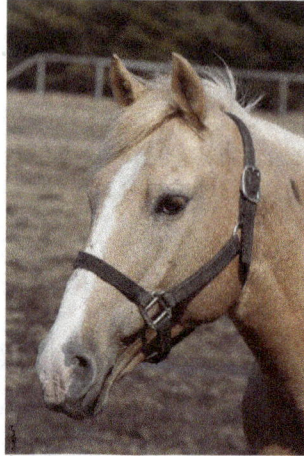

Horse wearing a nylon web halter (US) or headcollar.

Halters may be as old as the early domestication of animals, and their history is not as well studied as that of the bridle or hackamore. The word "halter" derives from the Germanic words meaning "that by which anything is held."

Uses

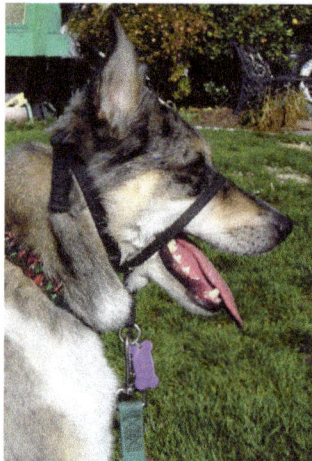

Dog wearing a halter-style collar.

A halter is used to lead and tie up an animal. It is used on many different types of livestock. Halters are most closely associated with Equidae such as horses, donkeys, and mules. However, they are also used on farm animals such as cattle and goats and other working animals such as camels, llamas, and yaks. Halters generally are not used on elephants or on predators, though there are halters made for dogs.

Halters are often plain in design, used as working equipment on a daily basis. In addition to the halter, a lead line, lead shank or lead rope is required to actually lead or tie the animal. It is most often attached to the halter at a point under the jaw, or less often, at the cheek, usually with a snap, but occasionally spliced directly onto the halter. A standard working lead rope is approximately 9 to 12 feet (2.7 to 3.7 m) long.

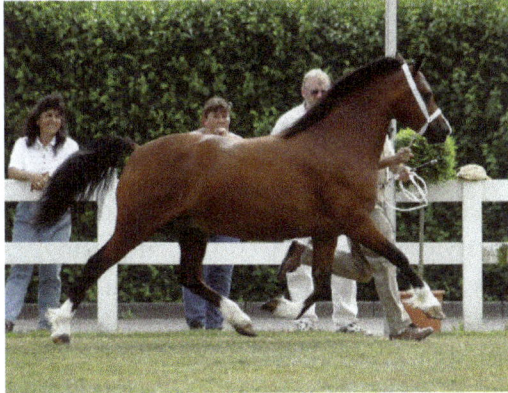
Horse shown in hand, wearing a Yorkshire halter.

However, specially designed halters, sometimes highly decorated, are used for in-hand or "halter" classes at horse shows and in other livestock shows. When an animal is shown in an exhibition, the show halter is fitted more closely than a working halter and may have a lead shank that tightens on the head so that commands from the handler may be more discreetly transmitted by means of the leadline. A shank that tightens on the animal's head when pulled is not used for tying the animal.

Halters are designed to catch, hold, lead and tie animals, and nothing else. However, some people ride horses using a halter instead of a bridle. In most cases, it is not safe to ride in an ordinary stable halter because it fits loosely and provides no leverage to the rider should a horse panic or bolt. It is particularly unsafe if the lead rope is used as a single rein, attached to the leading ring under the jaw.

Construction

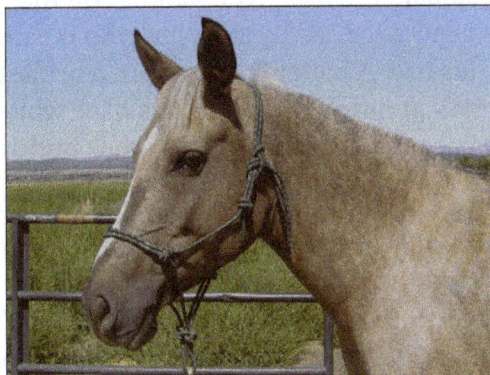
A rope horse halter

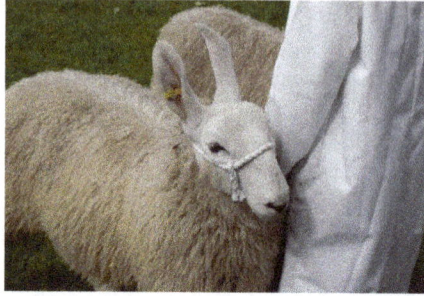

Sheep wearing a cotton rope halter.

Halters may be classified into two broad categories, depending on whether the material used is flat or round. Materials include cured leather, rawhide, rope, and many different fibers, including nylon, polyester, cotton, and jute. Leather and rawhide may be flat or rolled. Fibers may be woven into flat webbing or twisted into round rope. Flat or round dictates the construction method: flat materials normally are sewn to buckles or rings at attachment points; round materials are knotted or spliced. Knotted halters often are made from a single piece of rope.

Horse Halters

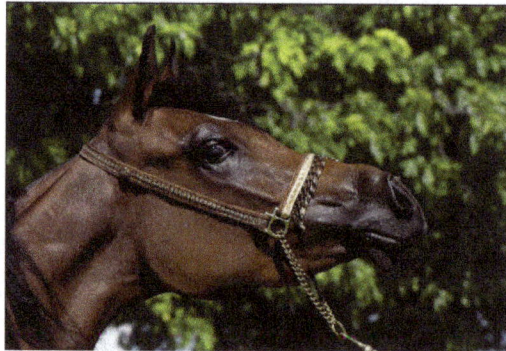

An Arabian horse in a stylized show halter

Horse halters are sometimes confused with a bridle. The primary difference between a halter and a bridle is that a halter is used by a handler on the ground to lead or tie up an animal, but a bridle is generally used by a person who is riding or driving an animal that has been trained in this use. A halter is safer than a bridle for tying, as the bit of a bridle may injure the horse's mouth if the horse sets back while tied with a bridle, and in addition, many bridles are made of lighter materials and will break. On the other hand, a bridle offers more precise control.

One common halter design is made of either flat nylon webbing or flat leather, has a noseband that passes around the muzzle with one ring under the jaw, usually used to attach a lead rope, and two rings on either side of the head. The noseband is usually adjusted to lie about halfway between the end of the cheekbones and the corners of the mouth, crossing over the strong, bony part of the face. The noseband connects to a cheekpiece on either side that go up next to the cheekbone to meet with a ring on either side that usually is placed just above the level of the eye. These rings meet the throatlatch and the crownpiece. The crownpiece is a long strap on the right-hand side of the halter that goes up behind the ears, over the poll and is buckled to a shorter strap coming up from the left. The throatlatch goes under the throat, and sometimes has a snap or clip that allows the halter to be removed in a manner similar to the bridle. Many halters have another short strap connecting the noseband and the throatlatch.

The halter design made of rope also has the same basic sections, but usually is joined by knots instead of sewn into rings. Most designs have no metal parts, other than, in some cases, a metal ring under the jaw where the lead rope snaps, or, occasionally, a recessed hook attachment where the crownpiece can be connected. However, in many cases, a loop is formed in the left side of the crownpiece and the right side of the crownpiece simply is brought over the horse's head, through the loop and tied with a sheet bend.

Leading

In addition to the halter, usually a lead (lead line, lead rope) or leash is used to lead or tie the animal. The lead is attached to the halter most often at a point under the jaw, less often at the cheek, and rarely above the nose. On horses, a lighter version of a headcollar or headstall is also used to attach a fly veil of waxed cotton strands or light leather strips onto a browband. Some fly masks are also made in a similar pattern to a headcollar and are often fastened with velcro tabs. These masks may also have ear and nose protection added to them. On both horses and dogs, halters may be used to attach a muzzle.

Safety and Security Issues

Steps in tying a safety slip knot on a lead rope

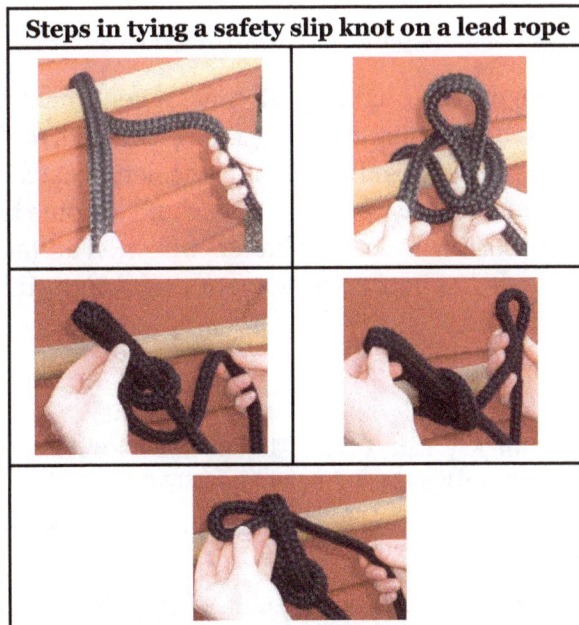

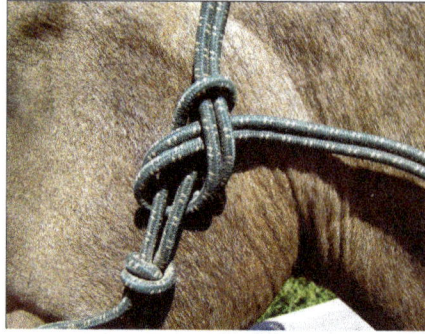

A modified sheet bend with the end falling away from the horse's head is used to secure a rope halter that lacks buckles

For tying, it is disputed if a halter should be made strong enough not to break under stress, or if it should give way when tension reaches a certain point in order to prevent injury to the animal. Usually the issue is of minimal concern if a tied animal is attended and the lead rope is tied with a slip knot that can be quickly released if the animal panics. However, in cases where a non-slip knot is tied, or if a soft rope is drawn tight and the knot cannot be released, or if the animal is left unsupervised, an animal panicking and attempting to escape can be seriously injured. Those who argue that the risk of injury is more of a concern than the risk of escape recommend halter designs that incorporate breakaway elements, such as a leather crownpiece, breakaway buckles, or easily detachable lead rope. Those who believe that escape is the greater danger, either due to concerns about escape or creating a recurring bad habit in an animal that learns to break loose that could become unable to be kept tied at all, recommend sturdy designs that will not break unless the handler deliberately releases a slipknot or cuts the lead rope. Between the two camps are those who recommend sturdy halters that will not break under normal pressure from a momentarily recalcitrant or frightened animal, but ultimately will break in a true panic situation, such as a fall.

Some users have the animal wear a halter at all times, even when stalled or turned out. Others have the animal wear a halter only when being led, held, or tied. The advantages of leaving a halter on are that the animal is often easier to catch. The disadvantages are that an animal may catch the halter on an object and become trapped or injured in some fashion. While experts advise leaving halters off when animals are turned out, if halters are left on unattended animals, breakaway designs that still will hold for everyday leading are recommended.

References

- Sylvia-Stasiewicz, Dawn; Kay, Larry (2010). The love that dog training program. Workman Publishers. p. 59. ISBN 9780761164074. Retrieved 26 February 2014.

- Beattie, William A. (1990). Beef Cattle Breeding & Management. Popular Books, Frenchs Forest. ISBN 0-7301-0040-5.

- Cottle, D.J. (1991). Australian Sheep and Wool Handbook. Melbourne, Australia: Inkata Press.

pp. 20–23. ISBN 0-909605-60-2.

- Diane Longanecker (2002). Halter-tying success: A Step-by-step Guide to Making Hand-tied, Rope Halters for Horses. William Eaton. p. 134. ISBN 9780963532060. Retrieved 2008-10-14.

- Carr, Shamar. Top 12 Things Your Dog Will Need and Love. Clinton Gilkie. Retrieved 26 February 2014.

- Baker, Andrew (1989). "Well Trained to the Yoke: Working Oxen on the Village's Historical Farms". Old Sturbridge Village. Retrieved May 2011.

- Bowers, Steve (Winter 2003–2004). "Draft Horse Shoeing... An Owner's Manual". Draft Horse Journal. 40 (4). Retrieved May 2011.

- Beck, Doug (Summer 1998). "Building a Shoeing Stock". The Small Farmer's Journal. Retrieved May 2011.

Various Veterinary Professions

Veterinary physicians are doctors who practice veterinary medicine by treating animals for their injury or disorders. They usually practice in clinics as well as in outdoors. Some of the other various veterinary professions are paraveterinary workers, equine dentists and animal nutritionists. The chapter explains to the readers the importance of the various veterinary professions.

Veterinary Physician

A veterinary physician, colloquially called a vet, shortened from veterinarian (American English, Australian English) or veterinary surgeon (British English), is a professional who practices veterinary medicine by treating disease, disorder, and injury in animals.

Description

In many countries, the local nomenclature for a veterinarian is a regulated and protected term, meaning that members of the public without the prerequisite qualifications and/or licensure are not able to use the title. In many cases, the activities that may be undertaken by a veterinarian (such as treatment of illness or surgery in animals) are restricted only to those professionals who are registered as a veterinarian. For instance, in the United Kingdom, as in other jurisdictions, animal treatment may only be performed by registered veterinary physicians (with a few designated exceptions, such as paraveterinary workers), and it is illegal for any person who is not registered to call themselves a veterinarian or prescribe any treatment.

Most veterinary physicians work in clinical settings, treating animals directly. These veterinarians may be involved in a general practice, treating animals of all types; they may be specialized in a specific group of animals such as companion animals, livestock, zoo animals or equines; or may specialize in a narrow medical discipline such as surgery, dermatology or internal medicine. As with other healthcare professionals, veterinarians face ethical decisions about the care of their patients. Current debates within the profession include the ethics of certain procedures believed to be purely cosmetic or unnecessary for behavioral issues, such as declawing of cats, docking of tails, cropping of ears and debarking on dogs.

History

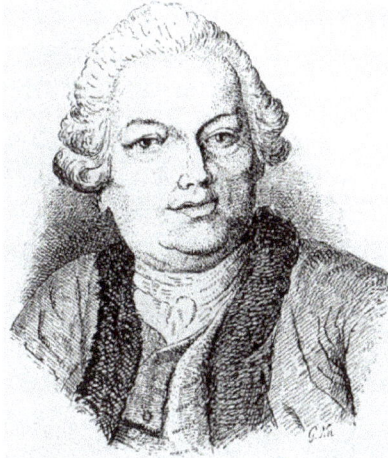

Claude Bourgelat established the earliest veterinary college in Lyon in 1761.

The first veterinary college was founded in Lyon, France in 1762 by Claude Bourgelat. According to Lupton, after observing the devastation being caused by cattle plague to the French herds, Bourgelat devoted his time to seeking out a remedy. This resulted in his founding a veterinary college in Lyon in 1761, from which establishment he dispatched students to combat the disease; in a short time, the plague was stayed and the health of stock restored, through the assistance rendered to agriculture by veterinary science and art."

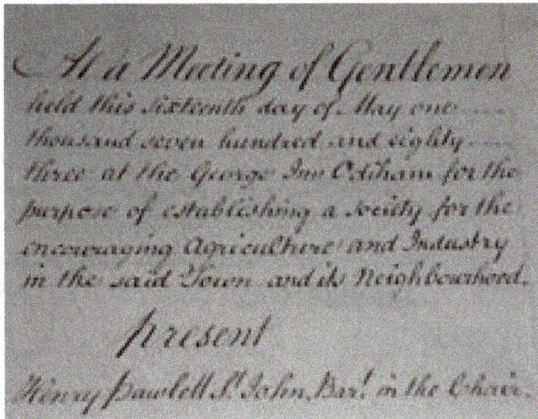

The Odiham Agricultural Society helped establish the veterinary profession in England.

The Odiham Agricultural Society was founded in 1783 in England to promote agriculture and industry, and played an important role in the foundation of the veterinary profession in Britain. A 1785 Society meeting resolved to "promote the study of Farriery upon rational scientific principles."

The professionalization of the veterinary trade was finally achieved in 1790, through the campaigning of Granville Penn, who persuaded the Frenchman, Benoit Vial de St.

Bel to accept the professorship of the newly established Veterinary College in London. The Royal College of Veterinary Surgeons was established by royal charter in 1844.

Veterinary science came of age in the late 19th century, with notable contributions from Sir John McFadyean, credited by many as having been the founder of modern Veterinary research.

Roles and Responsibilities

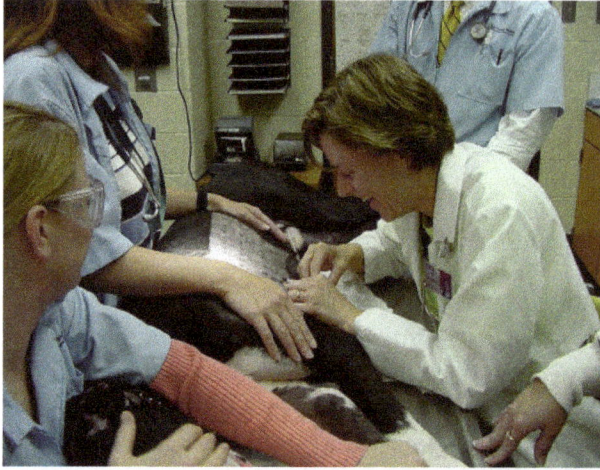

Veterinarians treat disease, disorder or injury in animals, which includes diagnosis, treatment and aftercare. The scope of practice, specialty and experience of the individual veterinarian will dictate exactly what interventions they perform, but most will perform surgery (of differing complexity).

Unlike in human medicine, veterinarians must rely primarily on clinical signs, as animals are unable to vocalize symptoms as a human would. In some cases, owners may be able to provide a medical history and the veterinarian can combine this information along with observations, and the results of pertinent diagnostic tests such as radiography, CT scans, MRI, blood tests, urinalysis and others.

Veterinarians must consider the appropriateness of euthanasia ("putting to sleep") if a condition is likely to leave the animal in pain or with a poor quality of life, or if treatment of a condition is likely to cause more harm to the patient than good, or if the patient is unlikely to survive any treatment regimen. Additionally, there are scenarios where euthanasia is considered due to the constrains of the client's finances.

As with human medicine, much veterinary work is concerned with prophylactic treatment, in order to prevent problems occurring in the future. Common interventions include vaccination against common animal illnesses, such as distemper or rabies, and dental prophylaxis to prevent or inhibit dental disease. This may also involve owner education so as to avoid future medical or behavioral issues.

Additionally veterinarians have important roles in public health and the prevention of zoonoses.

Employment

The majority of veterinarians are employed in private practice treating animals (75% of vets in the United States, according to the American Veterinary Medical Association).

Small animal veterinarians typically work in veterinary clinics, veterinary hospitals, or both. Large animal veterinarians often spend more time travelling to see their patients at the primary facilities which house them, such as zoos or farms.

Other employers include charities treating animals, colleges of veterinary medicine, research laboratories, animal food companies, and pharmaceutical companies. In many countries, the government may also be a major employer of veterinarians, such as the United States Department of Agriculture or the State Veterinary Service in the United Kingdom. State and local governments also employ veterinarians.

Focus of Practice

Veterinarians and their practices may be specialized in certain areas of veterinary medicine. Areas of focus include:

- Exotic animal veterinarian - Generally considered to include reptiles, exotic birds such as parrots and cockatoos, and small mammals such as ferrets, rabbits, chinchillas, and degus.

- Conservation medicine - The study of the relationship between animal and human health and environmental information.

- Small animal practice - Usually dogs, cats, and other companion animals/household pets such as hamsters and gerbils. Some practices are canine-only or feline-only practices.

- Laboratory animal practice - Some veterinarians work in a university or industrial laboratory and are responsible for the care and treatment of laboratory animals of any species (often involving bovines, porcine species, felines, canines, rodents, and even exotic animals). Their responsibility is not only for the health and well being of the animals, but also for enforcing humane and ethical treatment of the animals in the facility.

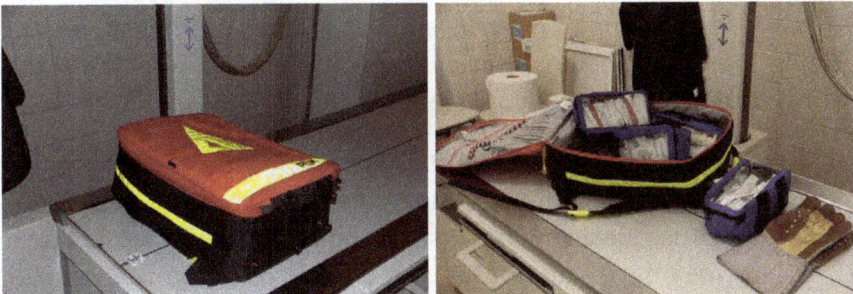

For on-call ambulance duty

- Large animal practice - Usually referring to veterinarians that work with, variously, livestock and other large farm animals, as well as equine species and large reptiles.

- Equine medicine - Some veterinarians are specialists in equine medicine. Horses are different in anatomy, physiology, pathology, pharmacology, and husbandry to other domestic species. Specialization in equine veterinary practice is something that is normally developed after qualification, even if students do have some interest before graduation.

- Food animal medicine - Some veterinarians deal exclusively or primary with animals raised for food (such as meat, milk, and eggs). Livestock practitioners may deal with ovine (sheep), bovine (cattle) and porcine (swine) species; such veterinarians deal with management of herds, nutrition, reproduction, and minor field surgery. Dairy medicine practice focuses on dairy animals. Poultry medicine practice focuses on the health of flocks of poultry; the field often involves extensive training in pathology, epidemiology, and nutrition of birds. The veterinarian treats the flock and not the individual animals.

- Food safety practice - Veterinarians are employed by both the food industry and government agencies to advise on and monitor the handling, preparation, and storage of food in ways that prevent foodborne illness.

- Wildlife medicine - A relatively recent branch of veterinary medicine, focusing on wildlife. Wildlife medicine veterinarians may work with zoologists and conservation medicine practitioners and may also be called out to treat marine species such as sea otters, dolphins, or whales after a natural disaster or oil spill.

- Aquatic medicine - mostly refers to veterinary care of fish in aquaculture (like salmon, cod, among other species), but can also include care of aquatic mammals. For certain countries with high economic income from aquaculture, this is an important part of the veterinary field (like Norway, Chile). Other countries (particularly those who are landlocked), might have little or no emphasis on aquatic medicine.

Veterinary Specialties

Veterinary specialists are in the minority compared to general practice veterinarians, and tend to be based at points of referral, such as veterinary schools or larger animal hospitals. Unlike human medicine, veterinary specialties often combine both the surgical and medical aspects of a biological system.

Veterinary specialties are accredited in North America by the AVMA through the American Board of Veterinary Specialties, in Europe by the European Board of Veterinary Specialisation and in Australasia by the Australasian Veterinary Boards Council. While some veterinarians may have areas of interest outside of recognized specialties, they are not legally specialists.

Specialties can cover general topics such as anesthesiology, dentistry, and surgery, as well as organ system focus such as cardiology or dermatology. A full list can be seen at veterinary specialties.

Mobile vs Stationary Practice

Some of the advantages of operating a mobile veterinary practice over a standard practice are the start-up and operating costs. Running a mobile practice is much less expensive than opening a brick and mortar location. A traditional physical location practice can cost upwards of $1,000,000 or more. A mobile vet can operate as low as $3000 for a box in an SUV to around $250,000 for a fully equipped custom built chassis. The advantages for the pet owner are less stress to their loved ones, less risk of disease transmission and convenience for having more than one pet all at close to the same cost as a clinic. Having to harness up or put a pet in a carrier to transport them to the clinic can be stressful to the animal. A 2015 study published in the Journal of American Veterinary Medical Association proved that blood pressure readings, pulse rates and body temperature rates were increased by 11-16% when those readings were done in the clinic versus in the home.

Salary

The mean salary for new graduates in the United States during 2010 was US$48,674, including nearly 50% going on to advanced study programs. Those not continuing their studies made US$67,359 at first, whereas veterinarians in the United Kingdom earned slightly less with new graduate wages at an average of £25,000.

The average income for private practice in the United States rose from $105,510 in 2005 to $115,447 in 2007. These increased values exceed those of public practice including uniformed services and government. In Australia, the profession wide average income was $67,000 in 2011 and this has declined compared to other professions for the past 30 years whilst graduate unemployment has doubled between 2006 and 2011.

Education and Regulation

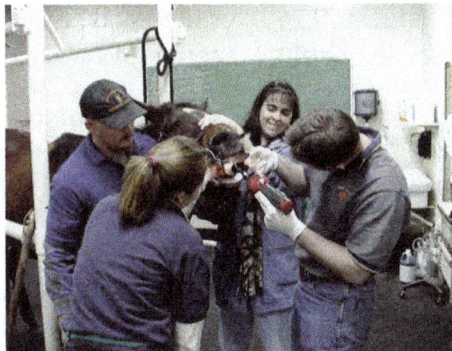

Veterinary students learning the dental treatment of a horse.

In order to practice, vets must complete both an appropriate degree in veterinary medicine, and in most cases must be registered with the relevant governing body for their jurisdiction.

Veterinary Science Degrees

Degrees in veterinary medicine culminate in the award of a veterinary science degree, although the title varies by region. For instance, in North America, graduates will receive a Doctor of Veterinary Medicine (Doctor of Veterinary Medicine or Veterinariae Medicinae Doctor; DVM or VMD), whereas in the United Kingdom or India they would be awarded a Bachelor's degree in Veterinary Science, Surgery or Medicine (BVS, BVSc, BVetMed or BVMS), and in Ireland graduates receive a Medicinae Veterinariae Baccalaureus (MVB). In continental Europe, the degree of Doctor Medicinae Veterinariae (DMV, DrMedVet, Dr. med. vet.) or Doctor Veterinariae Medicinae (DVM, DrVetMed, Dr. vet. med.) is granted.

The award of a bachelor's degree was previously commonplace in the United States, but the degree name and academic standards were upgraded to match the 'doctor' title used by graduates.

Comparatively few universities have veterinary schools that offer degrees which are accredited to qualify the graduates as registered vets. For example, there are 30 in the United States, 5 in Canada, and 8 in the United Kingdom (3 of which offer degrees accredited by the American Veterinary Medical Association (AVMA)).

Due to this scarcity of places for veterinary degrees, admission to veterinary school is competitive and requires extensive preparation. In the United States in 2007, approximately 5,750 applicants competed for the 2,650 seats in the 28 accredited veterinary schools, with an acceptance rate of 46%.

With competitive admission, many schools may place heavy emphasis and consideration on a candidate's veterinary and animal experience. Formal experience is a particular advantage to the applicant, often consisting of work with veterinarians or scientists in clinics, agribusiness, research, or some area of health science. Less formal experience is also helpful for the applicant to have, and this includes working with animals on a farm or ranch or at a stable or animal shelter and basic overall animal exposure.

In the United States, approximately 80% of admitted students are female. In the early history of veterinary medicine of the United States, most veterinarians were males. However, in the 1990s this ratio reached parity, and now it has been reversed.

Preveterinary courses should emphasize the sciences. Most veterinary schools typically require applicants to have taken one year equivalent classes in organic, inorganic chemistry, physics, general biology; and one semester of vertebrate embryology and biochemistry. Usually, the minimal mathematics requirement is college level calculus.

Individual schools might require introduction to animal science, livestock judging, animal nutrition, cell biology, and genetics. However, due the limited availability of these courses, many schools have removed these requirements to widen the pool of possible applicants.

List of AVMA Accredited Veterinary Colleges

School	State/Province or City	Country
Auburn University	Alabama	United States
Tuskegee University (probationary, 2013)	Alabama	United States
Midwestern University (provisional, 2013)	Arizona	United States
University of California	California	United States
Western University of Health Sciences (minor deficiency, 2012)	California	United States
Université de Montréal	Quebec	Canada
University of Calgary	Alberta	Canada
University of Guelph	Ontario	Canada
University of Prince Edward Island	Prince Edward Island	Canada
University of Saskatchewan	Saskatchewan	Canada
Colorado State University	Colorado	United States
University of Florida	Florida	United States
Murdoch University	Western	Australia
University of Melbourne	VIC	Australia
University of Sydney	NSW	Australia
University of Queensland	QLD	Australia
James Cook University	QLD	Australia
University of London	London	England
VetAgro Sup	Marcy l'Etoile	France
University College Dublin	Dublin	Ireland
Universidad Nacional Autonoma de México	Federal District	Mexico
Massey University	Palmerston North	New Zealand
The University of Edinburgh	Edinburgh	Scotland
University of Glasgow	Glasgow	Scotland
State University of Utrecht (minor deficiency, 2014)	Utrecht	The Netherlands
Ross University	St Kitts	West Indies
St. George's University (minor deficiency, 2011)	Grenada	West Indies
University of Georgia	Georgia	United States
University of Illinois	Illinois	United States
Purdue University	Indiana	United States
Iowa State University	Iowa	United States
Kansas State University	Kansas	United States

Louisiana State University	Louisiana	United States
Tufts University	Massachusetts	United States
Michigan State University	Michigan	United States
University of Minnesota (minor deficiency, 2014)	Minnesota	United States
Mississippi State University	Mississippi	United States
University of Missouri-Columbia	Missouri	United States
Cornell University	New York	United States
North Carolina State University	North Carolina	United States
The Ohio State University	Ohio	United States
Oklahoma State University	Oklahoma	United States
Oregon State University	Oregon	United States
University of Pennsylvania	Pennsylvania	United States
University of Tennessee	Tennessee	United States
Lincoln Memorial University (provisional, 2015)	Tennessee	United States
Texas A&M University	Texas	United States
Virginia Tech	Virginia	United States
Washington State University (minor deficiency, 2010)	Washington	United States
University of Wisconsin-Madison	Wisconsin	United States

Registration and Licensing

Following academic education, most countries require a vet to be registered with the relevant governing body, and to maintain this license to practice.

Dependent on where the vet practices (or wishes to practice), they may have to complete an examination or test in order to complete this registration. For instance, in the United States, a prospective vet must receive a passing grade on a national board examination, the North America Veterinary Licensing Exam. This exam must be completed over the course of eight hours, and consists of 360 multiple-choice questions, covering all aspects of veterinary medicine, as well as visual material designed to test diagnostic skills.

Postgraduate Study

The percentage electing to undertake further study following registration in the United States has increased from 36.8% to 39.9% in 2008. About 25% of those or about 9% of graduates were accepted into traditional academic internships. (2008 -696 graduates accepted a position in advanced study, 89.2% (621) accepted an internship (private practice, 74.5%; academic, 25.3%; and other internship, 0.2%). An additional 6.0% (42) accepted a residency). Approximately 9% of veterinarians eventually board certify in one of 40 distinct specialties from 22 specialty organizations recognized by the AVMA American Board of Veterinary Specialties (ABVS).

ABVS Recognized Veterinary Specialties

Anesthesiology and Analgesia	Animal Welfare	Avian Practice
Bacteriology\Mycology	Beef Cattle Practice	Behavior
Canine and Feline Practice	Canine Practice	Cardiology
Critical Care	Dairy Practice	Dentistry
Dermatology	Pharmacology	Poultry
Radiation Oncology	Radiology	Reproductive Medicine
Sports Medicine and Rehabilitation	Surgery	Swine Health Management
Toxicology	Virology	Zoological Medicine

Curriculum Comparison with Human Medicine

The first two-year curriculum in both veterinary and human medical schools are very similar in the course names, but at certain subjects relatively different in content. Generally, the more basal the field of science is (for example: biochemistry, biophysics, cell biology etc.), the more similar it is. Later on when the courses get more clinically oriented, more significant differences arise. Where some things are completely different, and other things are about the same. Considering the courses, the first two-year curriculum usually include biochemistry, physiology, histology, anatomy, pharmacology, microbiology, epidemiology, pathology and hematology.

Some veterinary school uses the same biochemistry, histology, and microbiology books as human medicine students; however, the course content is greatly supplemented to include the varied animal diseases and species specific differences. Many veterinarians were trained in pharmacology using the same text books as human physicians. As the specialty of veterinary pharmacology develop, more schools are using pharmacology textbooks written specifically for veterinarians. Veterinary physiology, anatomy, and histology is complex, as physiology often varies among species. Microbiology and virology of animals share the same foundation as human microbiology, but with grossly different disease manifestation and presentations. Epidemiology is focused on herd health and prevention of herd borne diseases, and foreign animal diseases. Pathology, like microbiology and histology, is very diverse and encompasses many species and organ systems. Most veterinary school have courses in small animal and also large animal nutrition, often taken as electives in the clinical years or as part of the core curriculum in the first two years.

The last two year curriculum of the two fields are similar only in their clinical emphasis. A veterinary student must be well prepared to be a fully functional animal physician on the day of graduation, competent in both surgery and medicine. The graduating veterinarian must be able to pass medical board examination and be prepare to enter clinical practice on the day of graduation, while most human medical doctors in the United States complete 3 to 5 years of post-doctoral residency before practicing medicine independently, usually in a very narrow and focused specialty. Many veterinarians do also complete a post-doctoral residency, but it is not nearly as common as it is in human medicine.

Impact on Human Medicine

Some veterinarians pursue post-graduate training and enter research careers and have contributed to advances in many human and veterinary medical fields, including pharmacology and epidemiology. Research veterinarians were the first to isolate oncoviruses, *Salmonella* species, *Brucella* species, and various other pathogenic agents. Veterinarians were in the forefront in the effort to suppress malaria and yellow fever in the United States. Veterinarians identified the botulism disease-causing agent, produced an anticoagulant used to treat human heart disease, and developed surgical techniques for humans, such as hip-joint replacement, limb and organ transplants.

In Popular Culture

Well-known depictions of a veterinarian at work are in James Herriot's series of books containing fictionalized stories of his career as a farm animal veterinarian in England, and the BBC's TV series *All Creatures Great and Small* based on the books.

The Three Lives of Thomasina starring Patrick McGoohan portrayed Andrew MacDhui a local veterinarian lives in a village in Scotland.

Doctor Dolittle is a series of children's books, one of which was turned into a 1967 movie. The movie was remade in 1998 with Eddie Murphy as Dr. Dolittle.

Hershel Greene from the popular series *The Walking Dead*, played by actor Scott Wilson is a veterinarian before turning his knowledge of medicine to treat human survivors and to study pathology of sick patients while in isolation during the time of the group's use of a prison as a fortified shelter.

US-based cable network Animal Planet, with animal-based programming, frequently features veterinarians. Two notable shows are *Emergency Vets* and *E-Vet Interns*, set at Alameda East Veterinary Hospital in Denver, Colorado.

The song *Grandma Got Run Over by a Reindeer*, performed by the husband and wife duo "Elmo & Patsy", is a song performed by a veterinarian, *Elmo Shropshire*, DVM.

Fictional character veterinarians in TV series and films include Steve Parker in *Neighbours*, Jim Hansen in *Providence*, and Vincent Ventresca in the horror film *Larva*.

In *Beethoven*, Dean Jones portrayed Dr. Herman Varnick, an evil veterinarian, with his associates Harvey and Vernon played by Oliver Platt and Stanley Tucci, who wanted all animals to be destroyed. They were foiled by the Newton Family and Beethoven. The Newton Family released other dogs from Dr. Varnick's captives.

Veterinary Malpractice

Most states in the US allow for malpractice lawsuit in case of death or injury to an animal from professional negligence. Usually the penalty is not greater than the value of the animal. For that reason, malpractice insurance for veterinarians is usually under $500 a year. Some states allow for punitive penalty, loss of companionship, and suffering into the award, likely increasing the cost of veterinary malpractice insurance and the cost of veterinary care. Most veterinarians carry much higher cost business, worker's compensation, and facility insurance to protect their clients and workers from injury inflicted by animals.

Criticisms

Concerns about the role of veterinary physicians in helping health threats survive and spread have been raised by several commentators, particularly with respect to pedigree dogs. Koharik Arman (2007) reached the following conclusion for example: "Veterinarians also bear some responsibility for the welfare situation of purebred dogs. In fact, the veterinary profession has facilitated the evolution of purebred dogs. 'Breeds' that would not normally be sustainable are propagated by the compliance of veterinarians to breeder wishes." This finding was echoed by Sir Patrick Bateson in his Independent Review of Dog Breeding following the broadcast of the BBC documentary *Pedigree Dogs Exposed*: "It's only the ready availability of modern veterinary medicine that has permitted some conditions...to become widespread."

Paraveterinary Workers

Paraveterinary workers are those people who assist a veterinary physician in the performance of their duties, or carry out animal health procedures autonomously as part of a veterinary care system. The job role varies throughout the world, and common titles include veterinary nurse, veterinary technician, veterinary assistant and veterinary technologist, and variants with the prefix of 'animal health'.

The scope of practice varies between countries, with some countries allowing suitably qualified paraveterinary workers a scope of autonomous practice, including minor surgery, whilst others restrict their workers to simple assisting of the veterinarian.

Nomenclature

Veterinary Nurse and Technician

In the majority of anglophone countries, paraveterinary workers with a formal scope of practice, and a degree of autonomy in their role, are known as a veterinary nurses. The primary exception to this is in North America, where both the United States and Canada refer to these workers as veterinary (or animal health) technicians or technologists.

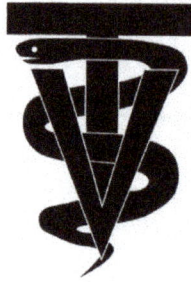

thumb

Human nursing associations have often claimed rights over the term 'nurse' and in some countries, this is protected by law. This was the case in the United Kingdom until 1984, where veterinary nurses were referred to as 'registered animal nursing auxiliaries', in line with the naming convention at the time for less qualified assistants in human nursing, called 'nursing auxiliaries'.

This is still the case in the United States, where the American Nursing Association and some state nursing associations have claimed proprietary rights to the term 'nurse'. Some veterinary technicians argue that as they spend approximately 90% of their time performing nursing tasks, they should be allowed to use the title of veterinary nurse, like their counterparts in other countries. Some argue that this is especially valid as their skill set is often greater than their human nursing counterparts, with the addition of skills such as radiology, laboratory work, pharmacy and more. Unofficially, many people (including vets and technicians) refer to these workers as veterinary nurses in conversation, as it is a succinct description of the role.

Veterinary Assistant

In most countries, a veterinary assistant is a person with fewer or no formal animal health qualifications, who has no autonomous practice, but who is designated to assist a vet and act under their direct instruction.

Training programs are often workplace-based, and no formal licence or certification is required to perform the role.

Local laws may restrict what activities a veterinary assistant may perform, as some procedures may only be legally completed by a registered practitioner, such as a vet or a veterinary nurse.

History

Veterinarians have had assistance from staff throughout their existence of the profession, but the first organised paraveterinary workers were the canine nurses trained by the Canine Nurses Institute in 1908, and announced in the magazine 'The Veterinary Student'. According to the founder they would "carry out directions of the veterinary surgeon, meet a genuine need on the part of the dog owners, and at the same time provide a reasonably paid occupation for young women with a real liking for animals".

In 1913, the Ruislip Dog Sanatorium was founded, and employed nurses to care for un- well dogs and in the 1920s, at least one veterinary surgery in Mayfair employed qualified human nurses to tend the animals. In the mid-1930s, the early veterinary nurses ap- proached the Royal College of Veterinary Surgeons for official recognition, and in 1938 the Royal Veterinary College had a head nurse appointed, but the official recognition was not given until 1957, first as veterinary nurses, but changed within a year to Royal Animal Nursing Auxiliaries (RANAs) following objection from the human nursing profession.

In 1951, the first formal paraveterinary role was created by the United States Air Force who introduced veterinary technicians, and this was followed in 1961 by a civilian programme at the State University of New York (SUNY) Agricultural and Technical College. In 1965 Walter Collins, DVM received federal funding to develop model cur- ricula for training technicians. He produced several guides over the next seven years, and for this work he is considered the "father of veterinary technology" in the United States.

In 1984, the term veterinary nurse was formally restored to paraveterinary workers in the United Kingdom.

Role and Responsibilities

Veterinary Technician Code of Ethics

1.Veterinary technicians shall aid society and animals by providing excellent care and services for animals.

2. Veterinary technicians shall prevent and relieve the suffering of animals with com- petence and compassion.

3. Veterinary technicians shall remain competent through commitment to life-long learning.

4. Veterinary technicians shall promote public health by assisting with the control of zoonotic diseases and educating the public about these diseases.

5. Veterinary technicians shall collaborate with other members of the veterinary medi- cal profession in efforts to ensure quality health care services for all animals.

6. Veterinary technicians shall protect confidential information provided by clients, un- less required by law or to protect public health.

7. Veterinary technicians shall assume accountability for individual professional actions and judgments.

8. Veterinary technicians shall safeguard the public and the profession against individuals deficient in professional competence or ethics.

9. Veterinary technicians shall assist with efforts to ensure conditions of employment consistent with the excellent care for animals.

10. Veterinary technicians shall uphold the laws/regulations that apply to the technician's responsibilities as a member of the animal health care team.

11. Veterinary technicians shall represent their credentials or identify themselves with specialty organizations only if the designation has been awarded or earned.

The scope of practice for paraveterinary workers varies by jurisdiction, and by qualification level. In some places, more than one grade of paraveterinary worker exists. For instance, in the United Kingdom there are both veterinary nurses, who are qualified professionals with a protected title, and veterinary assistants, who do not have a single level of qualification which they must attain, and whose title is not protected. Furthermore, job roles may be divided further into roles such as Veterinary Surgical Technician, Veterinary Emergency and Critical Care Technician, Veterinary Technician Anesthesia Specialist, etc.

At the higher levels, veterinary nurses or technicians may be able to practice skills autonomously, including examinations and minor surgery on animals, without the direct supervision of a veterinarian.

Paraveterinary workers are likely to assist the vet, or perform by themselves on behalf of the vet, medical skills such as observations (e.g. taking and recording pulse, temperature, respiration etc.), wound and trauma management (e.g. cleaning and dressing wounds, applying splints etc.), physical interventions (e.g. catheterizations, ear flushes and venipuncture) and preparing and analysing biological samples (e.g. performing skin scrapings, microbiology, urinalysis, and microscopy).

Dependant on their scope of practice and training, they may also be called upon to operate diagnostic screening equipment, including electrocardiographic, radiographic and ultrasonographic instruments, including complex machines such as computed tomography, magnetic resonance imagers and gamma cameras. In veterinary hospitals, veterinary technicians can perform complete blood counts, differential counts, and morphologic examinations of blood.

Paraveterinary workers would commonly assist veterinarians in surgery by providing correct equipment and instruments and by assuring that monitoring and support equipment are in good working condition. They may also maintain treatment records and inventory of all pharmaceuticals, equipment and supplies, and help with other administrative tasks within a veterinary practice such as client education.

Client education plays a key role of the veterinary technician's responsibilities to effectively communicate sometimes complex medical instructions in a positive and understandable way, and to facilitate the patient's care as an intermediary between the doctor, hospital and the patient. In this way, open lines of communication are established that can benefit the patient and hospital.

Education and Qualification

The level of education of a paraveterinary worker will depend on the role they are performing, and the veterinary medico-legal framework for the area in which they are working. Many areas employ veterinary assistants, who have a simple role to directly assist the vet under direction, and may hold no formal qualification or training, or have been trained on the job.

Higher level paraveterinary workers, such as veterinary nurses, veterinary technicians or veterinary technologists, who have a scope of autonomous practice which they are expected to perform without instruction, are likely to have both formal qualifications and in many jurisdictions will also require a formal registration with a monitoring body.

In countries where the role of paraveterinary workers is most advanced, the qualification required is likely to be based in higher education, such as in the United States or Canada where veterinary technicians must normally gain an associate degree at an institution recognised by the American Veterinary Medical Association or Canadian Veterinary Medical Association, and can choose to study for an extended period to gain a bachelor's degree (which in America may confer the title 'technologist', rather than 'technician'), or the United Kingdom, where veterinary nurses enter the profession through either a two-year diploma programme or through completion of a foundation degree or honours degree.

In almost all cases, regardless of the level of formalised training, a high level of practical experience is usually required prior to a student being fully qualified, which may be completed as part of their course, or during a post-qualification period. This may require maintenance of a log of all work completed, which may need to be signed by a supervising professional (such as the vet or senior member of the paraveterinary staff) to indicate competence. In some cases, such as in the United States, video records may be required of some procedures, which may then be examined by the awarding or registration body.

Many countries, including the United Kingdom, Canada, and parts of the United States, restrict some elements of practice, and may restrict use of the recognised name, to those people currently registered with an appropriate licensing body, meaning that it would be illegal for any person not on the register to represent themselves as a paraveterinary worker, or to perform some of the procedures that a licensed professional could. The precise details of these restrictions vary widely between legal areas, and neighbouring areas may have different policies, as is the case in the various states of the US.

This licensing body may have its own requirements for maintaining a registration, and those who hold the requisite academic qualification may still have to complete a further range of exams or tests to become registered. For instance, in the United States, most areas use the Veterinary Technician National Exam, and this will be used by the state licensing authority (such as a state veterinary medical association) to qualify an applicant to become a registered veterinary technician.

In some cases, those people who qualified before the introduction of formal academic qualification requirements may still be working as paraveterinary workers, and may still be entered on a required register through the use of grandfather rights. For instance, in some states of the US, people with a set number of years or hours of experience assisting a veterinarian could sit for the Veterinary Technician National Exam, however this route was phased out in 2011, and future candidates must have an academic qualification.

Specialty Certification

Beyond credentialing as a veterinary technician specialty certification is also available to technicians with advanced skills. To date there are specialty recognitions in: emergency & critical care, anesthesiology, dentistry, small animal internal medicine, large animal internal medicine, cardiology, oncology, neurology, zoological medicine, equine veterinary nursing, surgery, behavior, nutrition, clinical practice (canine/feline, exotic companion animal, and production animal sub-specialties) and clinical pathology. Veterinary Technician Specialists carry the additional post-nominal letters "VTS" with their particular specialties indicated in parentheses. As veterinary technology evolves more specialty academy recognitions are anticipated.

By country

- Paraveterinary workers in Australia
- Paraveterinary workers in Belgium
- Paraveterinary workers in Denmark
- Paraveterinary workers in France
- Paraveterinary workers in Ireland
- Paraveterinary workers in Italy
- Paraveterinary workers in Japan
- Paraveterinary workers in New Zealand
- Paraveterinary workers in Norway

- Paraveterinary workers in South Africa

- Paraveterinary workers in Sweden

- Paraveterinary workers in Switzerland

- Paraveterinary workers in Thailand

- Paraveterinary workers in Turkey

- Veterinary medicine in the United Kingdom

- Veterinary medicine in the United States

Global Presence

Attempts at professional solidarity resulted in the creation of the International Veterinary Nurses and Technicians Association (IVNTA) in 1993. Its members currently include Australia, Canada, Denmark, Finland, France, Germany, Ghana, Hong Kong, Ireland, Japan, Malta, Nepal, New Zealand, Norway, South Africa, Spain, Sweden, Switzerland, Thailand, Turkey, the United Kingdom, and the United States. In 2007 the Accreditation Committee for Veterinary Nurse Education (ACOVENE) was established in an attempt to standardize veterinary technology education throughout the European Union and to allow movement of veterinary nurses educated in one member nation to employment in another. On the specialty front, the Swiss-based organization VASTA (*Veterinär Anästhesie Schule für TechnikerInnen und ArzthelferInnen -- Veterinary Anaesthesia School for Technicians and Assistants*) is a six module year-long program that is approved by the Association of Veterinary Anaesthetists (AVA), the European College of Veterinary Anaesthesia and Analgesia (ECVAA), the International Veterinary Academy of Pain Management (IVAPM), and that has applied for RACE (Registry of Approved Continuing Education) approval in the United States ("Assistants" in the VASTA title refers to assistant or junior veterinarians and not to unqualified veterinary assistants). Its instructors include diplomates of the ECVAA, nurse anesthetists from the human medical field, neurologists, and veterinary physical therapists. It is currently offered in Germany, Austria, and the German-speaking regions of Switzerland. It has previously been offered in the French-speaking region of Switzerland but is currently on hiatus there due to low participation. Courses are planned for the US and the UK in 2012. Successful completion of the course results in the awarding of the post-nominal letters VAT (Veterinary Anaesthesia Technician).

Veterinary Specialties

A veterinary specialist is a veterinarian who specializes in a clinical field of veterinary medicine.

Most specialties require a 1-year internship or 2 years of clinical practice prior to beginning a residency of 3–4 years' duration. Most specialties require the resident to produce some academic contribution (often in the form of a scientific publication) in order to qualify to sit the certifying examination. Admission or entry into a Veterinary Specialty residency program is quite competitive in the United States and Canada. A veterinarian needs to complete a 1 year internship or, for some residency programs, have 2 years of clinical experience. A Veterinary Specialist may be consulted when an animal's condition requires specialized care above and beyond that which a regular veterinarian can offer. Many Veterinary Specialists require a referral in order to be seen. After treatment, a Veterinary Specialist may stay in close contact with the referring veterinarian to provide ongoing treatment suggestions and advice. Veterinary specialists may earn 2-3 times more than general practice veterinarians.

Specialties

- Anaesthesiology

- Animal behavior

- Animal welfare

- Birds (pet and ornamental)

- Bovine

- Canine

- Cardiology

- Clinical pathology

- Clinical pharmacology

- Dentistry

- Dermatology (veterinary dermatology)

- Diagnostic imaging (diagnostic imaging of animals)

- Equine

- Emergency and critical care (veterinary intensive care and veterinary emergency medicine)

- Feline

- Internal medicine

- Laboratory animal medicine

- Microbiology (veterinary microbiology; clinical microbiology of animals)

- Neurology and neurosurgery (veterinary neurology; veterinary neurosurgery)

- Nutrition

- Oncology (cancer in animals)

- Ophthalmology (veterinary ophthalmology)

- Parasitology

- Pathology (veterinary pathology)

- Poultry

- Preventive medicine

- Radiology (veterinary radiology)

- Reptile and amphibian

- Shelter medicine

- Sports medicine

- Surgery

- Theriogenology

- Toxicology

- Zoological medicine (includes zoo, wildlife, aquatics, and exotic pet species)

American Veterinary Medical Association

"A veterinary specialist, as recognized by the AVMA, is a graduate veterinarian who has successfully completed the process of board certification in an AVMA-recognized veterinary specialty organization (ie, board or college). To become board certified, a veterinarian must have extensive post-graduate training and experience and a credential review and examinations set by the given specialty organization."

The American Veterinary Medical Association recognizes the following 21 veterinary specialty organizations:

- American Board of Veterinary Practitioners

- American Board of Veterinary Toxicology

- American College of Laboratory Animal Medicine

- American College of Poultry Veterinarians

- American College of Theriogenologists

- American College of Veterinary Anesthesia and Analgesia

- American College of Veterinary Behaviorists

- American College of Veterinary Clinical Pharmacology

- American College of Veterinary Sports Medicine and Rehabilitation

- American College of Veterinary Dermatology

- American College of Veterinary Emergency and Critical Care

- American College of Veterinary Internal Medicine

- American College of Veterinary Microbiologists

- American College of Veterinary Nutrition

- American College of Veterinary Ophthalmologists

- American College of Veterinary Pathologists

- American College of Veterinary Preventive Medicine

- American College of Veterinary Radiology

- American College of Veterinary Surgeons

- American College of Zoological Medicine

- American Veterinary Dental College

Proposed Specialty Organizations

- American College of Animal Welfare

- American College of Veterinary Parasitologists

European Board of Veterinary Specialisation

The European Board of Veterinary Specialisation recognizes the following 23 veterinary specialty organizations:

- European College of Zoological Medicine

- European College of Animal Reproduction

- European College of Bovine Health Management

- European College of Equine Internal Medicine

- European College of Laboratory Animal Medicine

- European College of Porcine Health Management

- European College of Poultry Veterinary Medicine

- European College of Small Ruminant Health Management

- European College of Veterinary Anaesthesia and Analgesia

- European College of Animal Welfare and Behavioural Medicine

- European College of Veterinary Comparative Nutrition

- European College of Veterinary Clinical Pathology

- European College of Veterinary Dermatology

- European College of Veterinary Diagnostic Imaging

- European College of Veterinary Internal Medicine - Companion Animals

- European College of Veterinary Neurology

- European College of Veterinary Ophthalmologists

- European College of Veterinary Pathology

- European College of Veterinary Public Health

- European College of Veterinary Pharmacology and Toxicology

- European College of Veterinary Surgeons

- European Veterinary Dentistry College

- European Veterinary Parasitology College

Veterinary Dentistry

Veterinary dentistry is the field of dentistry applied to the care of animals. It is the art and science of prevention, diagnosis, and treatment of conditions, diseases, and disorders of the oral cavity, the maxillo-facial region, and its associated structures as it relates to animals.

In the United States, veterinary dentistry is one of 20 veterinary specialties recognized by the American Veterinary Medical Association. Veterinary dentists offer services in the fields of endodontics, oral and maxillofacial radiology, oral and maxillofacial surgery, oral medicine, orthodontics, pedodontics, periodontics, and prosthodontics. Similar to human dentists, they treat conditions such as jaw fractures, malocclusions, oral cancer, periodontal disease, and stomatitis and other conditions unique to veterinary medicine (e.g. feline odontoclastic resorptive lesions).

Some animals have specialist dental workers, such as equine dental technicians who conduct routine work on horses.

Overview

Most pet owners are not aware that their pet has an oral problem so an examination of the Oral Cavity Overview should form part of every physical examination. Oral examination in a conscious animal can only give limited information and a definitive oral examination can only be performed under general anaesthesia.It is important to examine the whole animal, even when the primary complaint is the mouth. Some dental diseases may be the result of a systemic problem and some may result in systemic complications. In all cases, dental procedures require a general anaesthetic so it is important to establish the cardiovascular and respiratory status and canine and feline physiological values of the patient to avoid risks or complications.

Pain originating from dental problems is very rarely recognized by owners or professionals. Seldom will an animal become anorexic due to a dental problem. The exception to this is in the case of severe soft tissue injury, for example chronic gingivostomatitis. In general dental pain is a chronic pain, and it is only after treatment that an owner reports how much better their pet is doing. Pain is often mistaken for a pet just getting old. Very few clients examine their pets' teeth unless they are carrying out daily home care, so actual dental problems often go unnoticed.It is important to recognize symptoms that may have a link to dental diseases such as a nasal discharge or external facial swellings. In some cases, dental patients may even present with what appear to be neurological symptoms.

The main signs of oral disease include :

- Halitosis

- Broken or discoloured teeth

- Changes in eating behaviour

- Rubbing or pawing at the face

- Ptyalism

- Bleeding from the mouth

- Inability or unwillingness to open or close the mouth

- Change in temperament

- Morbidity

- Weight loss

Equine Dentistry

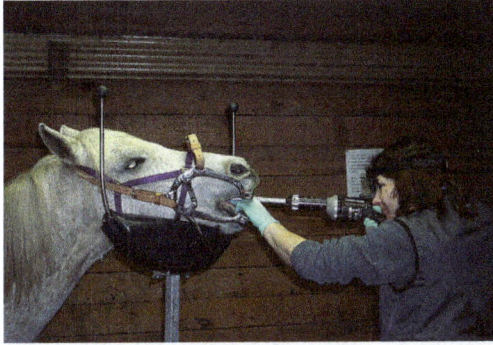

A veterinary physician performing dental work on a grey mare

Equine dentistry is the practice of dentistry in horses, involving the study, diagnosis, prevention, and treatment of diseases, disorders and conditions of the oral cavity, maxillofacial area and the adjacent and associated structures.

The practice of equine dentistry varies widely by jurisdiction, with procedures being performed by veterinary physicians (both in general and specialist practice), specialist professionals termed equine dental technicians or equine dentists, and by amateurs, such as horse owners, with varying levels of training.

In some jurisdictions, the practice of equine dentistry, or specific elements of equine dentistry, may be restricted only to specialists with specified qualifications or experience, whereas in others it is not controlled.

History

Equine dentistry was practiced as long ago as 600 BCE in China, and has long been important as a method of assessing the age of a horse. This was also practiced in ancient Greece, with many scholars making notes about equine dentistry, including Aristotle with an account of periodontal disease in horses, and in Rome with Vegetius writing about equine dentistry in his manuscript "The Veterinary Art".

In later years, the importance of dentition in assessing the age of horses led to veterinary dentistry being used a method of fraud, with owners and traders altering the teeth of horses to mimic the tooth shapes and characteristics of horses younger than the actual age of the equine.

The first veterinary dental school was founded in Lyon, France in 1762 and created additional knowledge about dentistry in horses and other animals.

Equine Dental Technicians

Equine dental technicians (also known colloquially as equine dentists, although this is not reflective of their official title) are veterinary paraprofessionals who specialise in routine dental work on horses, especially procedures such as rasping the sharp edges of teeth, also known as 'floating'.

Scope of practice may be dictated by statute. For instance, in the United Kingdom, any person, without any qualification may examine and rasp horses' healthy teeth with manual tools, remove deciduous caps (baby teeth) or remove supragingival calculus, whereas only qualified equine dental technicians or vets may remove teeth, rasp fractured teeth and use motorised dental instruments.

Relationship Between Vets and Lay Practitioners

There has been a long history of animosity between fully qualified vets and those lay people performing equine dentistry. This has led in some cases to an increase in voluntary and regulatory schemes in the sector. In the UK in the early 1990s, the veterinary profession engaged with lay practitioners to establish a formal system of examination and a register of qualified professionals. Whilst not compulsory, qualified persons were given an extended scope of practice for procedures normally reserved to vets.

In the United States, lay practitioners have been subject to legal action to gain injunctions against their practice, with case law in states including Missouri effectively precluding the practice of equine dentistry by persons other than vets.

Animal Nutritionist

An animal nutritionist is a person who specializes in animal nutrition, which is especially concerned with the dietary needs of animals in captivity: livestock, pets, and animals in wildlife rehabilitation facilities.

The science of animal nutrition encompasses principles of chemistry (especially biochemistry), physics, mathematics, ethology (animal behavior). An animal nutrition in the food industry may also be concerned with economics and food processing.

Education

A Bachelor of Science in agricultural, biological or related life sciences is usually required. A typical course would study metabolism of proteins, carbohydrates, lipids, minerals, vitamins and water, and the relationship of these nutrients and animal production. A Master's degree in nutrition is often seen in animal nutrition and the field often requires a Ph.D. in the science of nutrition.

Career Activities

Those with an educational background can expect to be employed in the following areas:

- Evaluating the chemical and nutritional value of various animal feeds, feed supplements, grass and forage for livestock, recreational animals such as horses and ponies, pet foods for companion animals, fish, and birds

- Nutritional disorders and the preservation of feeds

- Diet formulation and ration size

- Diets for performance and health

- Diets for reproduction of animals

- Economics of feeding systems

- Dietary regimens

- Animal studies and laboratory trials

- Marketing strategies for new food formulas

- Quality control and performance of feeds

- Investigating nutritional disorders and diet related diseases

Notable Animal Nutritionists

- Martin R. Dinnes, Ph.D.

- Mark Edwards, Ph.D.

- M. Steven Daugherty, Ph.D.

References

- McCurnin, Dennis M.; Bassert, Joanna M. (2006). Clinical Textbook for Veterinary Technicians, Sixth Edition. St. Louis, Missouri: Elsevier Saunders. p. inside front cover. ISBN 0-7216-0612-1.

- Tutt, Cedric (2007). BSAVA Manual of Canine and Feline Dentistry (BSAVA British Small Animal Veterinary Association (3rd ed.). UK: BSAVA. p. 200. ISBN 0905214870.

- "American Board of Veterinary Specialties". AVMA. American Veterinary Medical Association. Retrieved 12 December 2015.

- "Accredited Veterinary Colleges". AVMA. American Veterinary Medical Association. Retrieved 12 December 2015.

- "ABVS - Recognized Veterinary Specialty Organizations". AVMA.org. American Veterinary Medical Association. Retrieved 12 December 2015.

- "DVM Curriculum — College of Veterinary Medicine at Michigan State University". Cvm.msu. edu. 2009-12-07. Retrieved 2013-07-05.

- "Veterinarians : Occupational Outlook Handbook : U.S. Bureau of Labor Statistics". Bls.gov. 2012-04-26. Retrieved 2013-07-05.

- "Technologist vs Technician?". Canadian Association of Animal Health Technologists and Technicians. Retrieved 24 Jul 2011.

- "Policy Update Memo April 25, 2008: Veterinary Technician National Exam (VTNE) 2010 Eligibility Requirements" (PDF). American Association of Veterinary State Boards. Retrieved 24 Jul 2011.

- Bateson, Patrick (14 January 2010). "Independent Inquiry into Dog Breeding". Retrieved 16 January 2010.

Evolution of Veterinary Science

Hippiatrica is a collection of the ancient Greek texts that focus on the concern and care shown towards animals, horses in particular. Epizootic and mulomedicina chironis are the alternative topics explained in the chapter. The topics discussed in the section are of great importance to broaden the existing knowledge on the evolution of veterinary science.

Mulomedicina Chironis

The *Mulomedicina Chironis* (literally, "Chiron's Medicine for Mules") is a 4th-century medical treatise on medicine for treating horses, written in Latin.

Author

The name of the author is stated to be a certain Chiron Centaurus, which was certainly not the author's real name, but was likely a witty pseudonym.

Sources

The *Mulomedicina Chironis* lists several sources: Apsyrtus, Cato the Elder, Columella, Gargilius Martialis, and also some anonymous and lost writings. The book is not a translation of the Greek veterinary texts, the so-called Hippiatrica, although there's no denying the texts are useful to understand the *Mulomedicina*.

As a Model for Other Works

The *Mulomedicina Chironis* is the main source for Vegetius' *Mulomedicina*. The same Vegetius says at one point (Mul. 1, prologue 3-4): *Chiron vero et Apsyrtus diligentius cuncta rimati eloquentiae inopia ac sermonis ipsius vilitate sordescunt.* ("In spite of their care, Chiron and Apsyrtus don't sound good due to their poor expression and style error.")

Manuscripts

There remain two manuscripts containing the *Mulomedicina Chironis*. The first manuscript, the 15th century CLM 243, was found in 1885 at the Bavarian State Library in Munich by Wilhelm Meyer. The second manuscript, D III 34 dating from 1495) was discovered in 1988 at Basel University Library by Wener Sackmann.

Hippiatrica

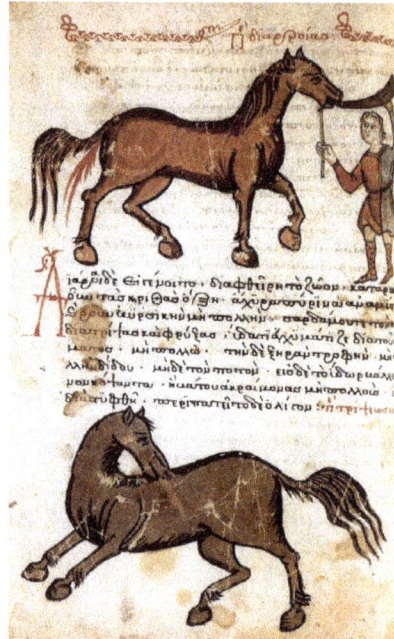

Folio from the *Hippiatrica* with written and illustrated instructions on drenching a horse to induce diarrhea.

The *Hippiatrica* is a Byzantine compilation of ancient Greek texts, mainly excerpts, dedicated to the care and healing of the horse. The texts were probably compiled in the 5th or 6th century AD by an unknown editor. Currently, the compilation is preserved in five recensions in twenty-two manuscripts (containing twenty-five copies) ranging in date from the 10th to the 16th century AD.

Contents

Seven texts from Late Antiquity constitute the main sources of the *Hippiatrica*: the veterinary manuals of Apsyrtus, Eumelus (a veterinary practitioner in Thebes, Greece), Hierocles, Hippocrates, and Theomnestus, as well as the work of Pelagonius, and the chapter on horses from the agricultural compilation of Anatolius. Although the aforementioned authors allude to their classical Greek veterinary predecessors (i.e. Xenophon and Simon of Athens), the roots of their tradition mainly lie in Hellenistic agricultural literature derived from Mago of Carthage. In the 10th century AD, two more sources from Late Antiquity were added to the *Hippiatrica*: a work by Tiberius and an anonymous set of *Prognoses and Remedies*. Content-wise, the sources in the *Hippiatrica* provide no systematic exposition of veterinary art and emphasize practical treatment rather than on aetiology or medical theory. However, the compilation contains a wide variety of literary forms and styles: proverbs, poetry, incantations, letters, instructions, prooimia, medical definitions, recipes, and reminiscences. In the entire *Hippiat-*

rica, the name of Cheiron, the Greek centaur associated with healing and linked with veterinary medicine, appears twice (as a deity) in the form of a rhetorical invocation and in the form of a spell; a remedy called a *cheironeion* is named after the mythological figure.

Epizootic

In epizoology, an epizootic is a disease event in a nonhuman animal population, analogous to an epidemic in humans. An epizootic may be: restricted to a specific locale (an "outbreak"), general (an "epizootic") or widespread ("panzootic"). High population density is a major contributing factor to epizootics. Aquaculture is an industry sometimes plagued by disease because of the large number of fish confined to a small area.

Defining an epizootic can be subjective; it is based upon the number of new cases in a given animal population, during a given period, and must be judged to be a rate that substantially exceeds what is expected based on recent experience (*i.e.* a sharp elevation in the incidence rate). Because it is based on what is "expected" or thought normal, a few cases of a very rare disease (like a TSE outbreak in a cervid population) might be classified as an "epizootic", while many cases of a common disease (like lymphocystis in esocids) would not.

Common diseases that occur at a constant but relatively high rate in the population are said to be "enzootic" (*cf.* the epidemiological meaning of "endemic" for human diseases). An example of an enzootic disease would be the influenza virus in some bird populations or, at a lower incidence, the Type IVb strain of VHS in certain Atlantic fish populations.

An example of an epizootic would be the 1990 outbreak of Newcastle disease virus in double-crested cormorant colonies on the Great Lakes that resulted in the death of some 10,000 birds.

Permissions

Index